MEDICINAL HERBS OF SANTA CRUZ COUNTY

Written and Illustrated by

Levi Glatt

FOREST ACADEMY PRESS * SANTA CRUZ, CA

Cataloging Data
Glatt, Levi.
Medicinal Plants of Santa Cruz County/by Levi Glatt.
Includes botanical illustrations and bibliographical references.
Artwork and book design by Levi Glatt.
First Edition.
ISBN- 978-1548723194

Published by:
Forest Academy Press
229 Forest Avenue
Santa Cruz, California 95062

Acknowledgements

I would like to thank Cheri Tuttle Callis, LAc, Acupuncturist and Herbalist, for valuable advice and suggestions throughout the researching process and for inspiring me to learn about medicinal plants in greater depth.

I would like to thank Dr. Darren Huckle, LAc., DAOM, and Herbalist, for answering my questions and giving valuable information from his vast experience and knowledge.

I would like to thank the entire Riekes Nature Awareness community for mentoring me over the years and awakening a deeper understanding and appreciation for the natural world. Riekes instructors taught me how to prepare salves, honey infusions, and more, for which I am grateful. I would like to thank Dylan Mathews for teaching me how to identify and prepare dozens of local plants and guiding me through breathtaking natural areas around Santa Cruz, many of which I had never before explored.

Last but not least, I wish to thank Rena Dubin for initially inspiring me about herbs, helping me prepare my first salves and tinctures, and accompanying me on my first plant harvesting expeditions. Thank you for your help with the proof-reading and editing stages of completing this book, and your advice, enthusiasm, and encouragement throughout this amazing journey.

DISCLAIMER

Medicinal Herbs of Santa Cruz County *is not intended as a guide for serious identification; rather, this book explains the exciting possibilities* **after** *a plant is successfully identified. Other field guides, which provide more detailed information and focus on identification, should be sourced for this crucial step. I suggest doing further research before experimentation. I am not responsible for your mistakes related to plant identification, preparation, or any choices made regarding the information in this book. Be smart, think realistically about your health, and take into account that specific herbs, or medicinal herbs in general, may not work for you. Seeking advice from a health care professional is always recommended.*

TABLE OF CONTENTS

INTRODUCTION

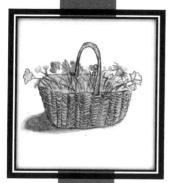

Since the origins of humanity, people have harmonized with plants and used them as a source of food. Gradually, as the human race continued to thrive, we began to understand that medicine, as well as food, could be derived from the leaves, roots, flowers, seeds, stems, bark, and fruits from specific plants. People administrated constant trial and error for tens of thousands of years to determine which herbs healed what ailments and how to properly prepare them to release the healing components. Besides experimentation, people most likely observed animals self-heal by eating specific plants.[1] Humans continued to fight against illnesses, by expanding their knowledge with medicinal herbs and passing on that knowledge through the generations. Early archeological evidence proves that plants have been used for healing in the Paleolithic Age, about 60,000 years ago.[2]

Traveling forward fifty-five thousand years brings us to the Sumerians, who wrote lists of herbs, and the ancient Egyptians, who also copiously researched herbs.[3] Many cultures throughout the world explored the healing side of plants, including the Ancient Greeks who, lucky for us, recorded their findings, and the Chinese, whose ancient practices serve as a foundation to this day.

Following in the footsteps of countless generations, we too can discover the wisdom of herbs. Wildcrafting local medicinal herbs is very satisfying, and creates a greater connection to the landscape. When you wildcraft your own healing remedies, you are not only infusing the herbal components, but are preserving the experience of harvesting to be reawakened with each use. For example, every time I consume my Aralia Honey Infusion, I remember the river bank, the consistency of the damp, pebbly soil, and the peaceful, shady stillness. Plants are a gift from the earth, and can be appreciated and used with gratitude.

Working with local herbs is also economical. While small quantities of herbal concoctions are sold at stores for high prices, particularly tinctures and syrups, homemade remedies can be manufactured for almost nothing, and are just as effective. A homemade quart of Blue Elderberry Tincture is cheaper than one ounce of the same tincture at a store.

Another advantage of working with local herbs is that they are fresh. Herbs bought in a store or online are, by necessity, dried. While working with dried herbs can be convenient and effective, many plants are more potent when fresh. Picking and processing local herbs can yield powerful products.

All the medicinal herbs in this book are local to Santa Cruz County, and most of them live in other regions of California and the world. No matter where you live, if you have access to any natural areas, there are bound to be medicinal plants. In addition to wildcrafting, other possible options are planting herbs in your garden or purchasing dried herbs from your local health food store.

The purpose of this book is to spread awareness and amazement towards these miraculous natural healers which share the planet with us. I hope that you will be inspired to discover the incredible healing magic the natural world has to offer, and observe more closely what many people walk past without a glance. The herbs in this book are only a small portion of the useful plants in Santa Cruz. I hope by reading this book you are motivated to do further research, since there is a lot more to be discovered. Happy herbal experimenting!

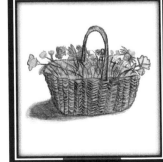

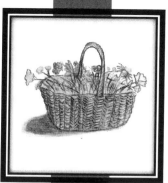

GUIDE TO HARVESTING HERBS FROM THE LANDSCAPE

Foraging from the landscape can be a perfectly sustainable practice; after all, humans have been gatherers since the beginning of our species. Although it may sometimes appear that gathering plants harms the environment, if done with respect, appreciation, and intention, foraging leaves little trace. Foraging gives a deep sense of gratitude for creation. Treating the earth like an untouchable museum prevents any opportunity for learning to be responsible caretakers of nature.[1]

IDENTIFYING PLANTS

I am always amazed with how many useful plants are visible, when one is in the habit of paying attention. Even in the most urban areas, such as sidewalk cracks and vacant lots, medicinal herbs can thrive. To successfully discover a new plant, begin by researching and learning about the species, with a focus on its appearance and characteristics. It is of utmost importance to fully identify plants before harvesting. Be careful and patient when collecting wild plants by never eating or preparing an herb until you are completely positive of its identity.[2] Although the consequences of consuming the wrong plants can be fatal, thorough identification can eliminate the risk of improper consumption.

Samuel Thayer in his book *Nature's Garden* explains the following steps to successfully identifying herbs:

The first step is to look at a field guide and see that it resembles the photograph. Most people stop here and think they have a proper identification.

However, if your intention is to consume this plant, you need to undergo the following steps. Read the description in order to verify that the specimen fits numerous characteristics, without mentally forcing it. Next, cross-reference your plant with multiple field guides. Find many specimens, since appearance can vary from plant to plant and in different seasons. After completing these steps, you should be familiar enough with the plant of interest to bet your life on it.[3]

Before harvesting, learn what parts are used, and the proper methods for preparation.[4] Even if one part of a plant is edible, all portions are not necessarily safe to use. **This book is not intended for serious identification; it explains the exciting possibilities *after* a plant is successfully identified.** Other field guides, which provide more detailed information and focus on identification, should be sourced for this crucial step.

Developing plant awareness and setting good intentions is the key to successful harvesting. With patience you will find the plant, an exciting first step. Once correctly identified for the first time, I guarantee that you will see the herb popping up in many other places, and eventually everywhere in the habitat. It is remarkable how increasingly easier it is to locate and identify an herb the more you try.

I believe that encountering a medicinal herb and then seeing it everywhere is due to a combination of the following ideas: the process of learning and developing awareness is enough to cause you to notice the plants; and by directing spiritual energy and setting good intentions, the land responds and directs one in the right direction. Exploring the magical world of plants and choosing specimens to harvest is a process that should be performed with respect and good intentions. As Nick Neddo says in his book *The Organic Artist*: "Take your time when hunting for materials on the landscape. Be patient with your pursuit and keep the image of what you want in your mind. Think of it as a conversation with the landscape."[5]

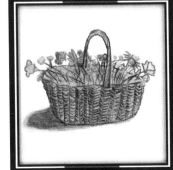

HARVESTING SUSTAINABLY

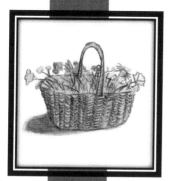

Harvesting herbs should come from a deep place of awe, gratitude, inspiration, and spiritual connection. You may want to meditate with the plant in its natural habitat for ten to twenty minutes in order to study, send positive energies, ask questions, harvest, and then thank the miraculous healer.

Do your best to harvest in a sustainable manner and in appropriate moderation, taking into account that your actions effect the population as a whole. Only take from a plant when there is a plentiful supply of the portions you wish to gather. If the flora does not appear healthy and thriving, picking may cause harm to its well-being. In addition, only pick when there are many specimens of each plant species in an area, especially when uprooting and taking an entire herb from the landscape. It is important to harvest in a way that minimally harms the plant and ecosystem. It is usually better to spread the forage amongst multiple plants instead of just one, although not always.

Gathering invasive plants, such as Himalayan Blackberry, can benefit the environment. The seeds and greens of most annual weeds can be gathered with little hesitation. In general, harvesting seeds or berries benefits the plant, so harvest as much as you want. If you feel inclined to give back, spread some of the seeds. The most vulnerable parts are the underground root systems, such as roots and bulbs. Make sure not to overharvest these, carefully taking only a small portion of the population. For plants that have larger root systems, portions can be collected with mindfulness.[6]

Even though it is tempting to over-pick, it is also important to only take what you are sure you will need and use. Michael Moore, in his book *Medicinal Plants of the Pacific West*, explains his experience with overharvesting: "Remember, know a few plants well, know what you will need, and don't try for the record number of shopping bags full of later unused (or in a year maybe unknown) dried herbs you bring back from a picking trip. I have held that record for twenty years—I warn and scold from experience."[7]

HARVESTING HAZARDS

CONTAMINATION

Many exciting weeds grow on roadsides, and are convenient for identification - it is amazing what you can observe when stopped in traffic! I mention roadside locations in the "Where to Find It" sections for identification purposes only. On roads and highways, pollution from cars results in contaminated vegetation. Additionally, major roads are usually sprayed with herbicides. Since the area has been sprayed, a four-foot portion borders major thoroughfares that is often visibly vacant of vegetation. The surviving greenery just outside of this herbicide line may contain toxic chemicals. **A minimum of fifty feet from roads is suggested for all herbal preparations.**

Additionally, contamination can occur when dogs or other animals pass through an area. I do not recommend harvesting herbs next to solid evidence that animals have passed through the area.

POISON HEMLOCK

Poison Hemlock (*Conium maculatum*) is a three-to-five foot high plant that grows in meadows and in partially-shaded regions near water. The stock is usually covered in purple spots and the leaf clusters are made up of tiny, serrated leaflets. Poison Hemlock's clusters of tiny white flowers[8] somewhat resemble Fennel, and the entire shrub looks similar to other wild plants. Poison Hemlock is one of North America's deadliest plants.[9] If any part is ingested, the consequences are fatal for humans and animals. Death can occur in only an hour or two, and there are no known antidotes.[10]

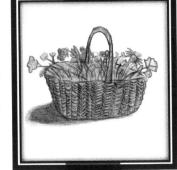

POISON OAK

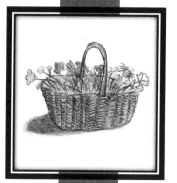

Western Poison Oak (*Toxicodendron diversilobum*) is a common, low-growing shrub that tends to entangle itself in brambles and trees. Western Poison Oak has sets of three shiny, coarsely scalloped leaves that are green in spring and early summer, red in autumn, and nonexistent in winter. Western Poison Oak thrives in shaded areas such as forests, but will also grow in partially shady habitats under trees.

When one brushes against the leaves and stems, an oil known as urushiol absorbs into the skin.[11] This causes a Poison Oak skin rash, also called contact dermatitis, with itching, bumps, and blisters. The best way to prevent Poison Oak rashes is to know how to identify this plant and therefore avoid contact.[12]

Although it is important to be aware of these hazards, this should not scare you away from gathering plants from the landscape. By properly identifying plants before harvesting, and avoiding Poison Hemlock, Poison Oak, and contaminated areas, you are ready to safely set out on wonderful herbal expeditions.

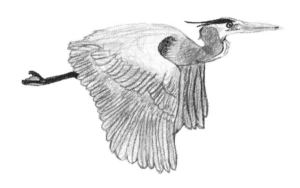

GLOSSARY OF HERBAL PREPARATIONS

For a detailed explanation of these preparations, see "Basic Internal Recipes" in "Recipes."

Infusion---herbs steeped in already boiled water, also known as "tea."

Decoction---herbs added to water and brought to a boil for 15 – 20 minutes. Ideal for tougher plant parts such as roots or bark, in contrast to tender leaves and flowers where an infusion is the best option.

Tincture---herbs steeped in alcohol for several weeks or months.

Vinegar---herbs steeped in vinegar for at least one month.

Syrups---a combination of an herbal decoction and raw honey.

Honey infusion---herbs directly infused in raw bee honey.

For a detailed explanation of these preparations, see "Basic External Recipes" in "Recipes."

Herbal oil---An infusion of herbs in oil.

Salve---an ointment made from herbal oil and beeswax.

Poultice---an herb paste for external application.

Compress---a cloth bandage saturated with a liquid herbal preparation.

Bath---an infusion of herbs in hot bathwater.

Soak---a bath delivered to only a specific area of the body.

Gargle/mouthwash---infusions, decoctions, or diluted tinctures gargled and swished around in the mouth.

Steam Inhalation---infusions and decoctions inhaled into the lungs.

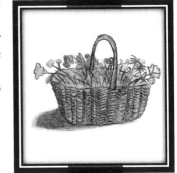

GLOSSARY OF HERBAL ACTIONS

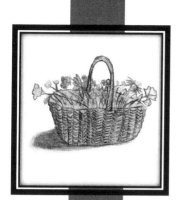

Analgesic---relieves pain, internal or externally.

Anti-bacterial---kills bacteria, which cures internal or external bacterial infections. Also known as an antibiotic.

Anti-viral---kills viruses, which cures internal or external viral infections.

Anti-fungal---kills fungi, which cures external or internal fungal infections.

Anti-microbial---kills micro-organisms in general, including bacteria, viruses, and fungi. Also known as an antiseptic.

Anti-inflammatory---reduces inflammation or swelling, externally or internally.

Anti-spasmodic---relieves involuntary muscle spasms, relaxing the body internally.

Anti-oxidant---contains molecules capable of stopping the damage of free radicals in the body. This can prevent oxidative stress such as cardiovascular diseases, inflammatory diseases, aging, cancer, and more.[1]

Astringent---causes the contraction of body tissues, which generally benefits the respiratory, urinary, and digestive tracts, as well as the skin.

Aromatic---having a pleasant and distinctive smell due to a high volatile oil content.

Carminative---relieves flatulence and bloating by lining and soothing the digestive tract.

Circulatory stimulant---increases blood circulation throughout the body.

Diaphoretic---induces perspiration. Causing the body to sweat excessively can lower fevers.

Expectorant---expels mucus from the respiratory tract and relieves irritation.

Hemostatic---staunches bleeding internally and externally, stopping hemorrhages.

Laxative---stimulates evacuation of the bowels, relieving constipation.

Nervine---calms the nerves without inducing drowsiness.

Sedative---induces sleep and calms the body.

Stomatic---helps the digestive tract.

Tonic---promotes general health and well-being, and/or restores, tones, and invigorates the body.

Vulnerary---assists in the healing of wounds by accelerating cellular growth.

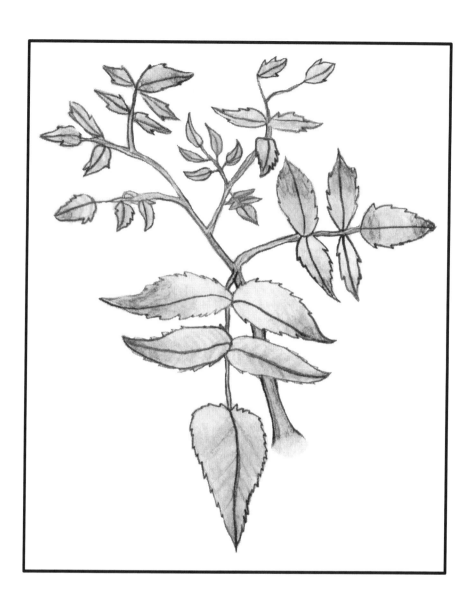

ARALIA

 Aralia californica

Aralia californica, *commonly known as Spikenard, is a bulky, three-to-six foot high perennial plant with serrated, horizontally positioned leaves that can grow to over a foot in length. Although one may expect this large plant to possess woody limbs, the branched stalks of Aralia are green. The leaves give off a spicy aroma when smashed. Beneath the soil lie the aromatic roots, which smell and taste spicy, sweet, and earthy. Smelling the roots make me imagine a cold day in wintertime. The flowers are clusters of green and white balls, resembling bursts of fireworks. The flower clusters develop into rich, black berries that prosper at the tops of each stalk in the autumn months.*

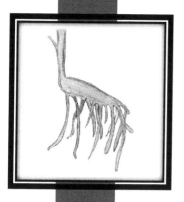

ARALIA:
SOOTHING THE
LUNGS AND THROAT

INTERNAL USAGE: *Aralia californica,* along with the greater known species *Aralia racemosa,* can be beneficial towards the common cold and can relieve dry and repeated coughs.[1] In addition, Spikenard can soothe sore throats, throat irritations,[2] bronchitis, and upper respiratory inflammations. Aralia is equipped with expectorant, anti-microbial, diuretic, and mildly astringent qualities.[3] Additionally, Spikenard can relieve urinary and gastrointestinal complaints such as cystitis and diarrhea,[4] as well as stress, thus calming the mind.[5]

EXTERNAL USAGE: Spikenard can be applied externally for wounds, cuts, and boils.[6] In addition, the root is topically anti-inflammatory, which can reduce herpes eruptions, eczema, and rashes such as contact dermatitis.[7] Additionally, the aroma can act as a flea repellent.[8]

PREPARATION: For internal preparation, the fresh roots can be made into a cough syrup with honey, and the roots, leaves, and berries can be tinctured or infused.[9] (See "Aralia Honey Syrup" in "Recipes.") If need be, simply chewing on the roots can keep the mouth moist and the lungs clear. Although spring and fall are best, the roots can be harvested year-round.[10]

For external properties, use a poultice,[11] dried root decoction, or diluted root tincture.[12]

WARNINGS: Do not use during pregnancy.[13]

Facts & Folklore

Aralia californica is native to California and Southern Oregon.[14] *Aralia californica's* close relative, *Aralia racemosa*, is an herb used since biblical times. Spikenard (*Aralia racemosa*) is an ancient herb, featured in the Ayurvedic healing customs of India,[15] referenced in Homer's *The Illiad*,[16] and in psalms attributed to King Solomon.[17] Spikenard was even one of the ingredients burned in the incense at the First and Second Holy Temples of Jerusalem more than 2,000 years ago.[18] Although Spikenard may seem like a funny sounding word, in Hebrew, Spikenard is "shebolet-nard", with "nar," meaning "light."[19] In Greek, the word for Spikenard means "pure and genuine."[20]

 # Where to find it

Aralia locates itself in shady, wet areas by creeks and riverbeds. In Santa Cruz County, Spikenard grows along Waddell Creek, Fall Creek, and forested creek beds in Felton and Bonny Doon. I have harvested Aralia roots in dried riverbeds at Little Basin and along the creek at Grey Whale Ranch, where it is quite abundant.

Aralia californica's close relative, *Aralia racemosa*, grows on the eastern half of the United States and Canada, and should not be harvested. *Aralia racemosa* is listed as "Special Concern" from the government's Natural Resources Conservation Service,[21] and is on the "To-Watch" list from United Plant Savers.[22] However, *Aralia californica* is abundant in Santa Cruz County. Although there are no rules regulating harvesting, do not take more than you need.

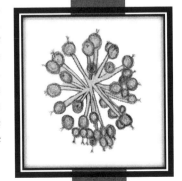

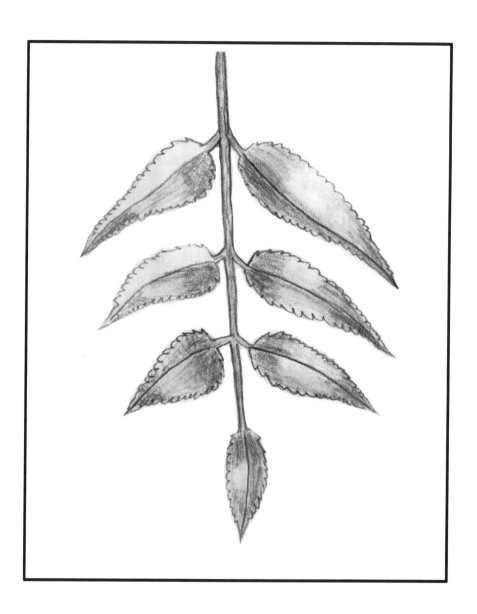

BLUE
ELDERBERRY

 Sambucus cerulea

Blue Elderberry grows from ten to thirty feet high, resembling a tree in California in contrast to the bush-sized shrubs of other regions. The limbs start near the ground and are arched, with the exception of some pencil-straight branches. The smaller twigs contain a starchy pith in the core. The leaves are serrated and pointed. There are usually seven to nine leaflets on each leaf cluster, always with a single leaf at the tip.

The flowers blanketing the tree in early summer are flat, star-shaped, fuzzy, yellow clusters. When the flowers ripen into rich, majestic berries, the Blue Elder tree teems with valuable goodness. The berries are in huge, flat clusters, weighing the branches downwards with ripe, copious wealth. These small berries are a light, pastel blue, although they reveal their purple-black radiance when polished.

BLUE ELDERBERRY: DEFENDING AGAINST COLDS AND INFLUENZA

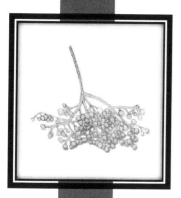

INTERNAL USAGE: Blue Elderberry can act as an extraordinary immune booster by increasing white bloodcells and releasing anti-inflammatory agents, cytokines,[1] vitamins A and C,[2] and anti-oxidant flavanoids into the body.[3] Blue Elderberry's immune boosting qualities fight against bacterial and viral infections, such as colds, influenza, sore throats, sinus infections, and bronchitis.[4] Additionally, the berries can reduce fever and eliminate chest and nose congestion from swollen mucus membranes.[5] In addition to the berries, the sweet Blue Elderberry flowers are also medicinal, and can aid in upper respiratory tract inflammations, and coughs, colds, or fevers due to diaphoretic properties.[6]

PREPARATION: Blue Elderberries can be prepared into a juice, decoction, syrup, or tincture, while Elder flowers should be made into an infusion. (See "Blue Elderberry Syrup" and "Blue Elderberry Tincture" in "Recipes.")

WARNINGS: The leaves, bark, stems, seeds, and unripe berries produce cyanide and possibly other toxins, and are poisonous in high concentrations.[7] When the *Sambucus cerulea* berries are ripe, they are technically non-toxic, although they should still be cooked before consuming.[8] Both Blue and Black Elderberry species (*Sambucus cerulea* and *Sambucus nigra*) have similar uses. Other Elderberry species, such as Red Elderberry, which also grows along the Central California Coast, require special preparation and may be poisonous to ingest.[9] Although this herb can be hazardous when prepared unwisely, like Samuel Thayer says in his book *Nature's Garden:*

"Don't let any of this talk about poisonous leaves and stems scare you away from the elderberry. After all, a bush so valuable has every right to protect itself. There are truly few plants that offer such diverse ways to be appreciated as the amazing elderberry." [10]

Facts & Folklore

Blue and Black Elderberries have been used in traditional medicine since the Middle Ages. [11, 12] In some folklore, the Elder tree is believed to host superhuman beings, while in other cultures, Elder is an herb of security, warding off witches and evil spirits.[13] Elder branches have been used to make instruments like the sambuke, a Greek word for an Elder flute, for which the genus *Sambucus* is named.[14] The berries, leaves, and bark can create colorful dyes,[15] such as the ones used by Native Americans for their basket designs.[16] Native Americans also crafted the straight shoots into arrows. [17]

 # Where to find it

Once I first identified *Sambucus cerulea*, I began seeing this tree everywhere in Santa Cruz County. If you are new to the Elder tree, the easiest time for identification is May through September, since the flowers and berries stand out against the green leaves. Blue Elderberry can be found along waterways, streams, mixed-forests, roadsides and in suburban areas.[18] I have wildcrafted Blue Elderberries at Felton Covered Bridge Park, spots off Graham Hill Road, and in neighborhoods. In addition, I have identified this magnificent tree at the Pogonip, off Glen Canyon Road, Mount Herman Road, on Freedom Boulevard near Aptos High School, Highway One near Watsonville, Mount Madonna Park, and Highway 129. Gather the Blue Elderberries in July through September. When picking the flowers, remember that you are preventing them from ripening into berries, and thus limiting the tree's future berry supply.

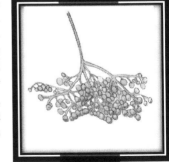

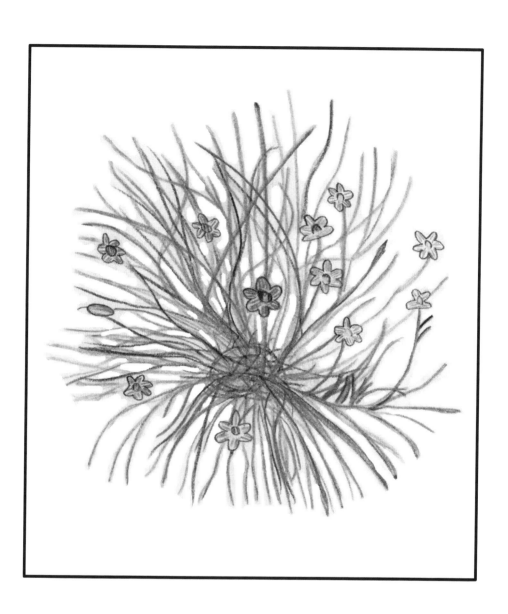

BLUE-EYED GRASS

 Sisyrinchium spp.

Blue-eyed Grass is a perennial herb that grows to around one foot in height. In winter, Blue-eyed Grass begins to produce cheery, bluish-purple flowers with six petals and bright yellow middles, or eyes, for which Blue-eyed Grass is named. Despite its name, Blue-eyed Grass is not actually a grass, but is in the iris family Iridaceae.[1] Blue-eyed Grass flowers seem to hover above the green, grassy tuft of spiky, pointed leaves. Individual flowers last only one day, but are produced in high quantities. The flowers mature into pods in June, exposing black seeds. Beneath the soil lies a fibrous root system.[2]

BLUE-EYED GRASS: CURING DIGESTIVE TRACT DISCOMFORTS

There are about seventy-five species of *Sisyrinchium* native to North and South America that are similar in appearance, and were used in identical ways.[3]

Although *Sisyrinchium* has been used extensively by Native Americans across the United States, the modern scientific research is limited.[4]

INTERNAL USAGE: Native Americans obviously considered this herb safe to use, since we know that they used Blue-eyed Grass to treat common disorders of the digestive tract, especially for children and elders.[5] Blue-eyed Grass was known to serve as a laxative.[6] The Ohlone tribe, native to Santa Cruz County, used the species *Sisyrinchium bellum* for indigestion and stomach pain,[7] while the California Coast Miwok tribe used *S. bellum* to soothe stomach aches.[8] In addition, the Cherokee people used the roots of other Blue-eyed Grass species for diarrhea and basic bowel regulation.[9]

Other uses of Blue-eyed Grass by Native Americans included easing menstrual disorders,[10] reducing fevers,[11] eliminating intestinal worms, and for birth control.[12]

PREPARATION: Blue-eyed Grass roots can be prepared into a decoction,[13] while the entire plant can be made into an infusion.[14]

WARNINGS: Modern scientific research is limited.

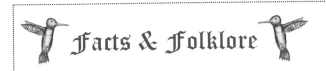

Facts & Folklore

Not only is Blue-eyed Grass a wild favorite, but this flower is also grown in gardens, where this plant is valued for its beautiful ornamental flowers and easy reproduction.[15] The leaves of Blue-eyed Grass are known to be edible when cooked. Native American tribes such as the Cherokee people cooked these leaves, consuming Blue-eyed Grass as a vegetable in spring mixes.[16]

 # Where to find it

After the first rain in winter, when the meadows and fields are lush and wet, Blue-eyed Grass can be found, thriving with its lively flowers. In Santa Cruz, you can find *Sisyrinchium* in many grassy, wild places, especially on grassy hills. This exuberant, cheery plant can be found in the Arboretum, UCSC meadows, Grey Whale Ranch, the Pogonip, and particularly Wilder Ranch, where these wildflowers thrive in astounding numbers.

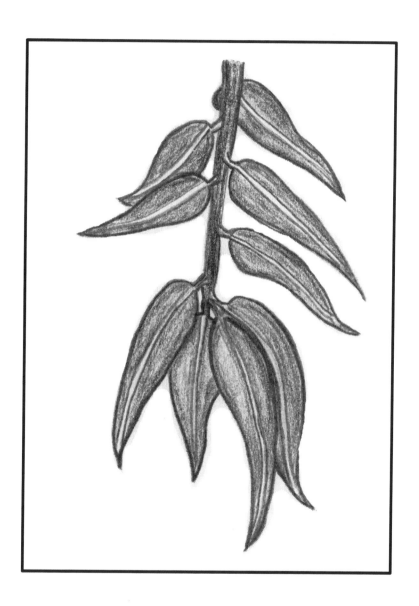

BLUE GUM EUCALYPTUS

 Eucalyptus globulus

Eucalyptus globulus *is a tall tree, about 100 to 180 feet high,[1] with thick, grayish-brown bark that peels off in long strips. Blue Gum Eucalyptus has sturdy, drooping branches that wave in the wind. The leaves covering those branches are dark green, usually crescent shaped, and pointed at the ends. The leaves are waxy, dotted, and textured. The strong, spicy scent they give is carried in the breeze. The sturdy seedpods of Blue Gum Eucalyptus are brown and intricate, with multiple slits at the top, forming a geometric, flower-like pattern.*

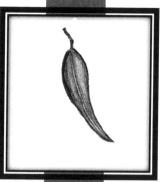

BLUE GUM EUCALYPTUS: CLEARING MUCUS AND SOOTHING THE LUNGS

INTERNAL USAGE: Blue Gum Eucalyptus is a popular cold remedy, mainly because this tree's leaves are anti-microbial and have expectorant qualities. Blue Gum Eucalyptus' expectorant properties can expel mucus from the lungs, ease bronchial congestion, and clear the nasal passages.[2] Blue Gum Eucalyptus can also reduce respiratory tract infections, coughs, whooping cough, asthma,[3] and sinus infections.[4]

E. globulus can also act as an astringent, anti-inflammatory, and mild antispasmodic.[5] This tree may also treat gallbladder and liver issues,[6] bladder infections,[7] throat inflammation,[8] ulcers, diabetes, flu symptoms, and fevers.[9] The leaves are known to possess insect repellent properties.[10]

EXTERNAL USAGE: Blue Gum Eucalyptus can treat minor wounds, burns, skin ulcers,[11] and acne,[12] as well as mouth and throat inflammations.[13] In addition, *E. globulus* has analgesic properties, ideal for muscle soreness and arthritis.[14]

PREPARATION: For the respiratory qualities to be released, the fresh or dried leaves should be infused. One should drink the resulting infusion or inhale the steam into the lungs. I have found the dried leaves, not fresh, to be the most potent when infusing in water. (See "Blue Gum Eucalyptus Steam Inhalation" in "Recipes.") Other internal preparations of *E. globulus* include tinctures, lozenges, and syrups.[15]

Externally, one should prepare a wash, compress,[16] bath, herbal oil,[17] or balm.[18]

WARNINGS: Consume internally and apply to the skin with caution, since the bark, leaves, and especially the oil are toxic in high doses.[19] Any consumption of the oil is not advised for pregnant or nursing women, children, or infants.[20]

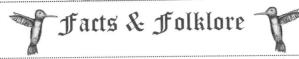

Facts & Folklore

Eucalyptus globulus appears a harmless and beautiful tree that is intrinsic to this region's habitat. This is a disguise. I have grown up in Santa Cruz without realizing how destructive this invasive tree has been to California. Eucalyptus originated in Australia, and was introduced to Europe in 1770. Decades later, as Eucalyptus spread throughout the world, the interest of many California settlers peaked.[21] Eucalyptus thrived in California. Everyone believed that Eucalyptus was valuable because it made great lumber, fuel, medicine, and wood pulp. The California settlers were excited that Eucalyptus grew quickly, and in harsh conditions.[22] However, Eucalyptus did not meet any expectations. Settlers soon discovered that Eucalyptus took seventy-five to one hundred years to become proper hardwood. If harvested earlier, it split, decayed, and rotted, and was not even suitable for fence posts or railroad track ties.[23] The bark was also extremely flammable, resulting in much destruction.[24] After millions of acres of Blue Gum Eucalyptus were planted, this tree destroyed the local ecosystem. Eucalyptus leaves and bark are toxic, so the native animals couldn't process the tree, as Australian animals were previously adapted to digest it.[25] They were driven out, along with the local plant species. Eucalyptus has severely altered the native landscape of California.

Where to find it

Blue Gum Eucalyptus is vastly distributed around Santa Cruz County, growing everywhere. At Natural Bridges and Lighthouse Field, Eucalyptus is enjoyed by monarch butterflies and people, while the cluster at the Upper Santa Cruz Yacht Harbor hosts a variety of seabirds, including Black-Crowned Night Herons and Great Blue Herons. At any spot in Santa Cruz County, you are guaranteed to find a Blue Gum Eucalyptus planted in your field of vision, either close or in the distance. Even though this tree is quite abundant, finding a location with accessible leaves can prove challenging. For convenient harvesting, look for low-hanging branches, and, if possible, pick fresh, young leaves off newer saplings. Some of my favorite places to pick the leaves include La Fonda Avenue near Harbor High School, Frederick Street Park, DeLaveaga, and Arana Gulch.

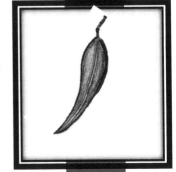

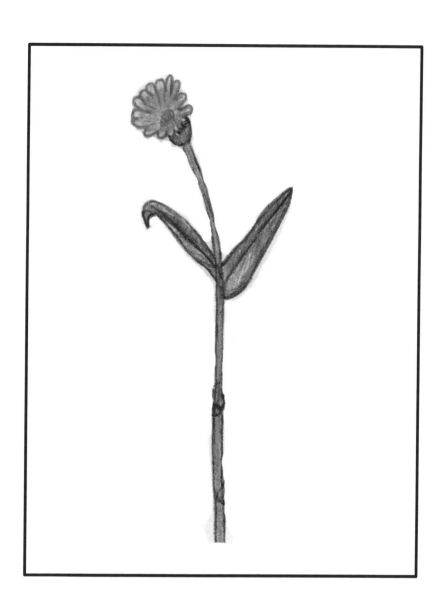

CALENDULA

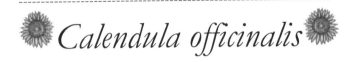

Calendula officinalis

Despite being a cheery garden favorite, Calendula officinalis *also appears in Santa Cruz as a "garden-escaped" volunteer. Calendula's vivid, orange flowers are sticky with a spicy aroma, and quickly produce in large quantities. The one to three foot high garden-escaped variety of Calendula has many tiny flowers, each with one or two rings of petals. In contrast, the tidy, gardened type has larger flowers with multiple rings of petals, just bursting with color. Calendula flowers mature into bizarre, green, alien-like seed heads. Since the "untamed" flowers are more sensitive to sunlight than the neat garden flowers, I have only seen them open from around 10:00 am - 2:00 pm.*

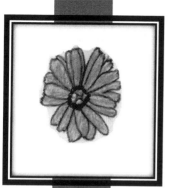

CALENDULA: RELIEVING INFLAMMATION

EXTERNAL USAGE: *Calendula officinalis* is one of the best known herbs for skin healing,[1] since the flowers are potent in topical herbal remedies,[2] as well as the leaves if needed. Calendula is an astringent,[3] antimicrobial and anti-inflammatory skin herb.[4]

When applied externally, Calendula can sustain healthy skin by reducing wounds, including cuts, burns, boils, bruises, sprains, skin ulcers,[5] insect bites and stings, [6] irritation, and infection.[7]

INTERNAL USAGE: Calendula can possess inflammation-related internal uses. Calendula can soothe inflammation of the lungs, mucus membranes, lymph nodes, tonsils,[8] mouth, throat, gums, and gastrointestinal tract. [9]

Calendula can reduce fevers, colds, flu, cramps, stomachaches,[10] ulcers, and nausea.[11] *Calendula officinalis* may also assist in detoxification, blood circulation, and menstrual cycle[12] and immune system regulation.[13]

PREPARATION: For external usage, Calendula flowers can be prepared into an infusion, tincture, poultice or compress.[14] My favorite preparation, however, is an herbal salve. Calendula flowers work miracles in a salve or balm, especially in combination with the herbs Yarrow and Plantain. (See "All Purpose Salve" in "Recipes.") An infusion of the preferably dry flowers should be created for internal purposes.[15]

WARNINGS: No known cautions.

Facts & Folklore

Calendula flowers are edible, but not particularly tasty in large quantities due to the sticky, bitter substance on the petals. Calendula has been incorporated into foods, such as syrups, breads, cheeses,[16] salads,[17] soups, and stews, mostly for color, but also to enhance the flavor[18] and garnish dishes.[19] The flowers are also employed as a dye in cosmetics and the cloth industry.[20] Calendula in Latin means "little clock" or "little calendar,"[21] named by the Romans because this herb can bloom nonstop and on the first day of every month of the calendar.[22] Since Calendula symbolizes happiness and exuberance, this herb was grown in order to spread joy.[23] The abundance of bright Calendula flowers resulted in frequent, worldwide usage.[24] In India, Calendula flowers decorated the Hindu statues,[25] glorified temple altars,[26] and even crowned the gods and goddesses.[27] The Ancient Egyptians believed Calendula had special rejuvenating powers.[28] Calendula petals were used by the Persians and Greeks for garnishing and flavoring food,[29] and by the Romans and Greeks in ceremonies featuring Calendula garlands.[30] Calendula has also been incorporated in Arabic,[31] Mayan, Aztec, and European traditions.[32] Recently, in the American Civil War, and later World War I, Calendula's wound-healing flowers were used on the battle grounds as emergency aid.[33]

Where to find it

Every winter and spring, volunteer Calendula grow abundantly in meadows and other open areas with any type of soil. In California, Calendula is a self-seeding annual, but can also exist as a shortly-lived perennial plant.[34] In any case, Calendula will seed abundantly, spreading quickly over an available area.[35] I have seen Calendula growing on the side of Highway 1, at Wilder Ranch, and in UCSC, specifically around the Life Lab, as well as open areas around the base of campus. Calendula can also be found growing in many yards, gardens, and suburban areas of Santa Cruz, even if not initially desired. It is interesting how the untamed variety of Calendula is a common weed, while the gardened version, also known as Pot Marigold, is a favorite ornamental flower.

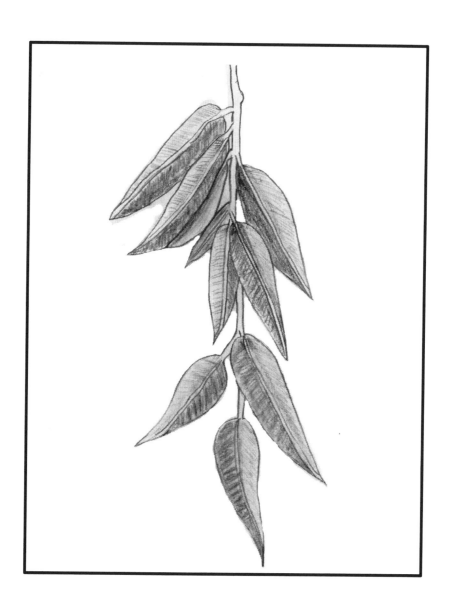

CALIFORNIA BAY

 Umbellularia californica

Growing up to one hundred feet tall,[1] California Bay, also known as California Laurel, is a medium-sized evergreen tree with widely spread, dense branches. The leaves are pointed at the tips and have distinct midribs. Each leaf holds an extremely strong spicy scent that is distinctive and carries well in the breeze. When the California Bay leaves yellow and fall, they sprinkle across the forest floor like a golden layer of sparkle. Umbellularia californica *produces bay nuts in autumn that are edible when roasted. The nuts fall to the ground encased by a purple-red flesh. The nuts and the flesh are tasty at first, but have a bitter aftertaste.*

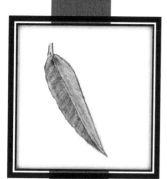

CALIFORNIA BAY: ANTI-SPASMODIC AND ANTI-FUNGAL

INTERNAL USAGE: As an anti-spasmodic, *Umbellularia californica's* leaves can relieve diarrhea, intestinal knots,[2] gas, and colic pain.[3] Consuming the leaves can relieve pain from migraines,[4] other types of headaches, and stress.[5] Because California Bay is also an astringent, this plant can assist in healing stomach ulcers.[6] California Bay's medicinal uses are due to concentrated volatile oils. By simply using California Bay in food, this plant will release many beneficial minerals, including calcium, iron, copper, manganese, selenium, potassium, zinc, and magnesium.[7] The leaves also have diuretic and appetite stimulant properties.[8]

EXTERNAL USAGE: *Umbellularia californica* is useful externally as well. California Bay has antimicrobial, and most specifically antifungal, skin cleansing properties. As an anti-fungal, California Laurel can cure types of tineas such as athlete's foot, ringworm, and jock itch.[9] Arthritis, muscle, and joint pain can also be cured with *Umbellularia californica*, primarily from a bath or a soak.[10] A momentary tingling sensation may be experienced when applying this herb upon the skin.[11] Inhaling the strong scent from the leaves or leaf tincture can effectively arouse someone who is feeling weak or dizzy.[12]

PREPARATION: It is preferable that the leaves are prepared fresh when using medicinally, as the volatile oils degrade quickly as they dry when in direct sunlight. Storing California Bay for medicinal use is possible, but somewhat complicated, as an airtight container in cool, dark conditions is required.[13] For internal use, infuse or tincture the fresh leaves. For external use, infuse the fresh leaves directly into hot bathwater, or add the tincture. The tincture can be saturated into a cotton swab to directly release its external uses onto the skin.[14]

WARNINGS: *Umbellularia californica's* actual leaves should not be consumed, as they may injure the digestive system and cause choking.[15] Pregnant women should avoid internal use of this plant, although infrequent culinary use is fine.[16] As I've experienced, deep inhalation of the leaves can cause sinus headaches[17] and sneezing,[18] although both symptoms dissipate within a few minutes.

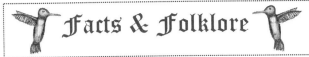

The origin of the Bay Laurel tree occurs in a myth featuring the sun god Apollo in Greek Mythology (the Mediterranean species, *Laurus nobilis*). When Apollo laid eyes upon a nymph named Daphne whom he instantly loved, he chased after her, but she did not love him back.[19] Apollo was physically gaining upon Daphne, when her pleas were answered and she was transformed into the first Bay Laurel tree.[20] Since Apollo could never wed Daphne, he honored her forever by adorning himself in a Laurel wreath, and using Laurel wood for lyres and arrows.[21] The Laurel wreath became a symbol of protection,[22] wisdom, peace,[23] and achievement, and was worn by army generals, rulers, and athletes in Ancient Greece.[24] Apollo protected this tree, using his powers of immortality to make the leaves eternally green.[25]

Umbellularia californica was sacred to the Kashaya Pomo people, a Californian tribe native to Sonoma County.[26] The leaves were rubbed on hunters' bodies to ensure a successful hunt, burned in the home to repel evil fortune, and waved over travelers as they departed.[27] California Bay nuts were roasted and used in jewelry by some California tribes. California Bay has very flexible wood and saplings, ideal for projects such as bow and arrow wild-crafting. Bay leaves are commonly used for culinary purposes, flavoring soups, stews, meats, sauces, rice, vegetables, and countless other delicious foods.[28]

 # Where to find it

California Bay trees grow inside redwood and riparian forests, and form forests of their own. I have noticed that these native trees tend to thrive on mountain slopes. In our ecosystem, I have identified California Bay at Henry Cowell, Big Basin, Rancho Del Oso, Gray Whale, Arana Gulch, the Pogonip, and forested UCSC regions. Be aware that gathering local Bay leaves for flavoring foods will have excessive potency when compared to those you may get in the store. You may want to use less California Bay leaves in your recipes since they will be more fresh and this variety is stronger.[29] Although autumn and winter are fine for gathering, spring and summer are the most ideal seasons, as the leaves are fresh and exuberant and the oils are strong.[30] Avoid using leaves infected with fungus and in other ways diseased.[31]

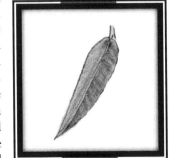

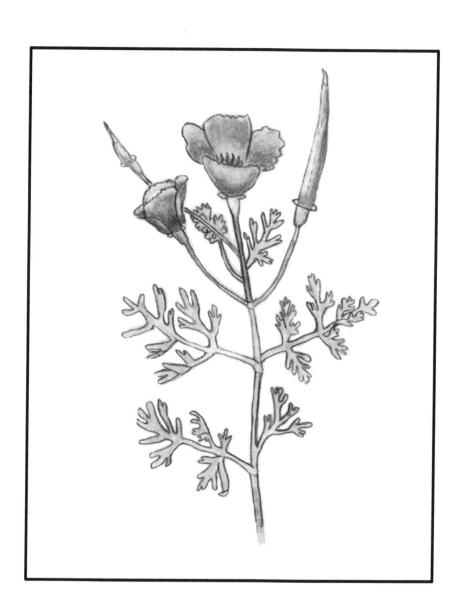

CALIFORNIA POPPY

 Eschscholzia californica

California Poppy is a joyful, native, annual wildflower that grows up to two feet in height. Eschscholzia californica *is famous for its bright orange four-petaled flowers. The uniquely shaped, intricate leaves are lacy and feathery, with many flat stems that branch from the base. When the petals fall, the flower middles develop into long and skinny seed pods. Orange colored juice usually bleeds out of the roots when cut. Although this plant looks delicate in appearance, it is quite invasive and disease-resistant.*

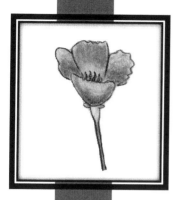

CALIFORNIA POPPY: RELAXING THE BRAIN AND NUMBING THE BODY

INTERNAL USAGE: California Poppy tea or tincture can greatly improve one's sleep, being a sedative in large doses. In lower doses, this poppy can reduce anxiety, which can relieve nervous tension and lower stress.[1] Additionally, California Poppy can treat headaches and has anti-spasmodic effects, which can cure nerve pain and joint or muscle symptoms.[2] The bitter qualities of the tincture can soothe the digestive tract and immune system. Internally and externally, the roots have an analgesic effect, healing pain and tension with a pleasant feeling afterwards.[3]

EXTERNAL USAGE: The juice from the root can be applied to any tooth pain for direct relief.[4]

PREPARATION: The entire plant, especially the fresh roots, should be tinctured. (See "California Poppy Tincture" in "Recipes.") The aerial parts can also be infused.[5]

WARNINGS: Do not take California Poppy if pregnant, nursing, or taking prescription medication.[6] California Poppy is related to *Papaver somniferum*, or opium poppy; although *Eschscholzia californica* has completely different components than opiates, it is chemically similar enough to test positive on a urine-based drug test.[7]

Facts & Folklore

Eschscholzia californica is native throughout the western United States, but is especially copious in California.[8] In 1903, this herb became California's state flower. When Spanish settlers came to California, they were awestruck when they saw abundant displays of these poppies lighting up the hills and coastal prairies, and they could even guide their ships by the sight.[9] Spanish settlers called this wild flower "Copa de Oro" which means "Cup of Gold." They also named the California coast "Land of Fire" after the bright displays of these orange wildflowers.[10] The unusual and hard to pronounce Latin name *Eschscholzia californica* was derived from Dr. Eschscholtz, a German naturalist in the early 1800s.[11]

 # Where to find it

California Poppies grow wild in any open field, meadow, or garden with full sun and any degree of soil. In Santa Cruz, the meadows and fields containing California Poppies include the Pogonip, UCSC meadows, Arana Gulch, and Wilder Ranch. In spring, California Poppies make the fields and meadows explode with color, especially when they mix with the blue lupines. Since California Poppy is the state flower, harvesting in the wild is considered an offense, although there are no legal regulations regarding the picking of this plant.[12]

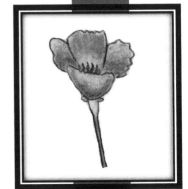

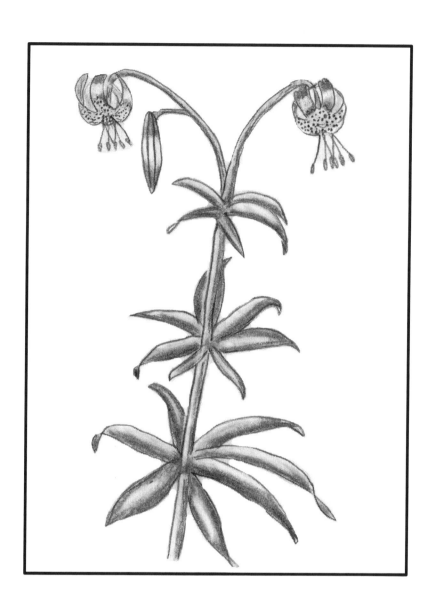

CALIFORNIA TIGER LILY

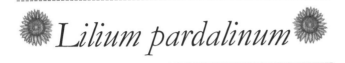

Lilium pardalinum

California Tiger Lily has a three to five foot high stalk with dark green, pointed leaves that fan out in whorls. The stem branches at the top, where magnificently beautiful buds and flowers hang downwards, blooming from May until July. The lily flowers are a bright orange-yellow color and are covered with dark spots, suggesting the name "Tiger Lily." The petals are typically curled back to reveal long stamen with dark, pollen-covered tips.

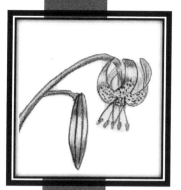

CALIFORNIA TIGER LILY: WOMEN'S HERB

INTERNAL USAGE: *Lilium pardalinum* is traditionally a woman's herb. Because of its anti-inflammatory nature, this herb can relieve vaginal inflammation, painful menstruation, menopausal symptoms, fibroids, and pelvic pains. In addition, California Tiger Lily can relieve uterine-neuralgic pain and the nausea and vomiting resulting from pregnancy.[1] California Tiger Lily can aid in urinary disorders such as urinary tract infections.[2]

California Tiger Lily may also cure problems of the heart, such as palpitations, pain,[3] and irregular heartbeat.[4] California Tiger Lily has been known to alleviate coughs and sore throats.[5] Due to this flower's pleasant scent, a steaming cup of California Tiger Lily can be used for depression, stress, boosting one's mood, and calming aggression.[6]

PREPARATION: California Tiger Lily can be prepared into a soup, infusion, or tincture, made from the entire fresh plant.[7]

WARNINGS: Tiger Lilies are extremely toxic to cats. Consumption by cats may result in kidney failure or even death. Ingesting the pollen is extremely toxic to humans.[8] Some subspecies are federally listed as endangered.[9]

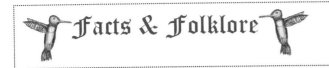

Facts & Folklore

Lilium pardalinum is native to California and southern Oregon. Tiger Lilies are commonly grown in gardens, since they don't require much water once fully grown and they look very ornamental. Tiger lilies are actually a family of flowers that once grew wild in many parts of the world.[10] However, many people uprooted Tiger Lilies and took them home for their own use, causing them to be an endangered species in some places.[11] Some subspecies have also been squeezed out by development.[12] Tiger Lily tubers, shoots, and buds are edible cooked and were eaten by Native Americans.[13] In Asia, the local Tiger Lilies are used in soups and recipes.[14]

 # Where to find it

California Tiger Lilies love very wet soils, which is why I have identified this plant along creekbeds. California Tiger Lily can grow along the shady banks of rivers, creeks, and ditches in Santa Cruz County. Since some subspecies are federally listed as endangered,[15] consider cultivating this scarce but beautiful herb for personal use instead of wildcrafting.

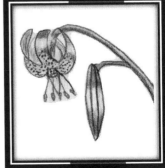

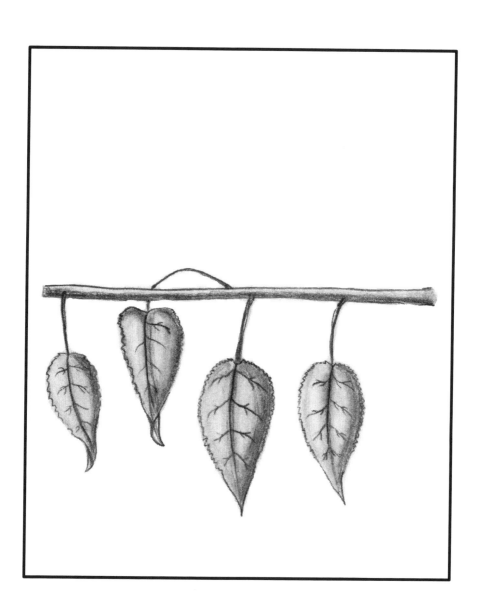

COTTONWOOD

Populus trichocarpa

The Cottonwood tree can grow up to one hundred feet in height, with high branches and thick bark. However, there are many young, miniature Cottonwoods in Santa Cruz that are around ten to fifteen feet high, these being the easiest to appreciate and use. Populus trichocarpa *is a pleasure to observe year-round. In winter or early spring, after the golden yellow leaves have fallen from the trees, buds form on every bare branch. Although called buds, they are not actually flower buds, but the beginning of leaves and leafy branches. These buds are coated in a sticky medicinal resin that smells strong, kind of like earthy, piney, sweet sap. It gets all over your fingers when gathered! The buds open up quickly into light green, heart-shaped leaves that are waxy and shiny from their sticky beginning. As the leaves grow rougher and darker, the Cottonwood tree reproduces by long and fluffy catkins that carry the seeds in the wind. The abundant white fluff feels like cotton, giving Cottonwood its name.*

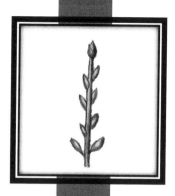

COTTONWOOD: REPAIRING THE SKIN AND RELIEVING PAIN

The Cottonwood tree's sticky spring buds teem with medicinal resin.

INTERNAL USAGE: Historically, Cottonwood was consumed for its internal uses, including coughs, chronic bronchitis, and lung congestion in tincture form.[1]

EXTERNAL USAGE: Nowadays, however, the fresh, resinous buds are more commonly used in a salve, also known as **Balm of Gilead.** Balm of Gilead is used externally for cuts, scrapes, burns, bruises, sore muscles, swelling, skin inflammation, arthritis, tissue damage,[2] sunburn,[3] and general pain-relieving and anti-microbial qualities.[4] I love gifting Balm of Gilead because this salve has been so helpful to many recipients. Friends and relatives have been grateful for Cottonwood's ability to heal broken capillaries due to aging, bruising, temporary pain, and skin damage. This pleasantly scented herb is one of the best known natural medicines in this region of the world.[5]

PREPARATION: Use the fresh, resinous buds in a salve. Preparing the oil can prove a challenging process, so please see "Balm of Gilead" in "Recipes." Just packing the fresh, resinous buds on the inflicted area directly may also heal these ailments if necessary.[6]

WARNINGS: No known cautions.

Facts & Folklore

Cottonwood was one of the most sacred trees to Native Americans, who believed that when the leaves rustled, they were speaking powerful words.[7] Because of the great height of Cottonwood, this majestic tree was thought to be connected to the sky and bring spiritual conduct down to earth.[8] Cottonwood is a very soft wood and is therefore great for many woodworking projects and crafts.

 # Where to find it

Cottonwood trees grow in open areas, usually near a water source. My favorite place to harvest Cottonwood in Santa Cruz is the Arboretum, where small trees grow plentifully along with their taller neighbors. However, I have also seen Cottonwood along the San Lorenzo River, other river and creek beds, and on the sides of many roads, especially Highway 129, where they are abundant and large.

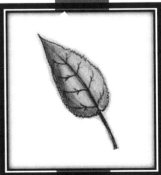

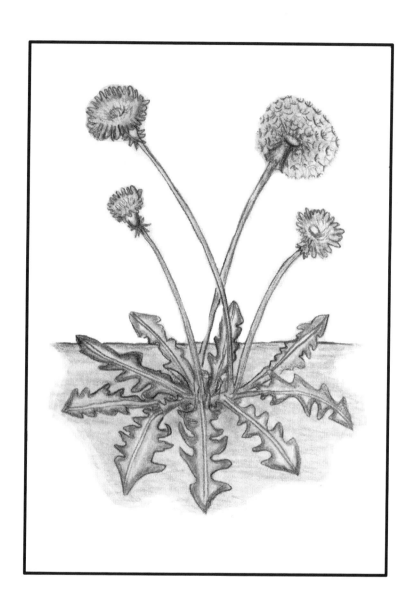

DANDELION

🌼 *Taraxacum officinale* 🌼

Dandelion is a low-growing perennial weed with bright, cheery yellow flowers that possess many rings of small petals. Once these colorful flowers turn to seed, they transform into white balls of fluff. When these balls are blown, the seeds scatter in the wind, which I have always found irresistible. The tall, juicy stems on which the flower and seed heads rest contain a white, bitter, milky substance. Towards the base of this plant are the leaves. Dandelion originated from the French word, "dent de lion," meaning "lion's tooth," referring to the jagged, deeply notched, toothed leaves.[1] Dandelion leaves, along with other parts of the plant, are edible, although with a bitter flavor. Dandelion leaves are eaten in salads and are in most packaged green mixes. The roots are dark brown, and filled with the same bitter, milky substance inside the stems. Dandelion is packed with vitamins A, B, C, and D, as well as the minerals iron, zinc, and potassium.[2]

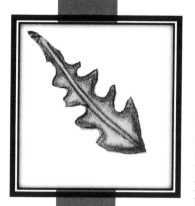

DANDELION: DIURETIC AND DIGESTION HELPER

INTERNAL USAGE: *Taraxacum officinale* roots and leaves can benefit the digestive system by stimulating the appetite, calming heartburn, burping, gas, and bloating,[3] and acting as a mild laxative.[4] Dandelion can act as an excellent diuretic, helpful for urinary disorders, liver problems (including jaundice), and gallbladder or kidney issues.[5] As a diuretic, Dandelions might help lower blood pressure, and may also lower cholesterol, normalize blood sugar, and help with diabetes and anemia.[6]

EXTERNAL USAGE: The milky substance in Dandelion is antimicrobial, astringent, and detoxifying, treating skin irritations such as eczema, ringworm, itching, and acne when one applies the milky juice to the area directly.[7]

Dandelion can also treat stiff and arthritic joints, sore muscles, and rough, chapped skin.[8]

PREPARATION: Fresh or dried Dandelion leaves and roots can be made into a tincture, decoction, juice extract, or capsule.[9] The fresh or dried flowers can be made into a salve.[10]

WARNINGS: People with kidney problems, gallbladder problems, or gallstones should consult their doctors before eating dandelion.[11] Rashes may occur for some people who are allergic to other members of the Asteraceae family.[12] Dandelions may interact with specific medications and drugs in a harmful way, so consult your health care professional.[13]

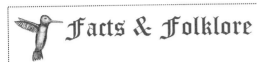

Facts & Folklore

Because Dandelion is bright and cheery, and has been used for food and traditional medicine in Mexico, North America, and China, the myths encompassing this herb are numerous and positive.[14] For example, Dandelion is known to bring hope, happy unions, good luck for the married couple, and answers to deep questions.[15] Dandelions have also been thought to increase psychic abilities and call spirits. Blowing on the Dandelion seed head to scatter the seeds has been proclaimed to bring love and affection to a loved one and grant wishes.[16] Dandelions were brought over to America from Europe in the early days of our country, where they spread across the entire continent quite rapidly.[17]

Where to find it

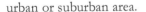

Dandelions will plant themselves in the open areas of Santa Cruz, from gardens, empty lots, grass lawns, and even sidewalk cracks, to more natural locations such as meadows and fields. Additionally, Dandelions live on the rocky banks of partially shaded or sunny rivers. Dandelions may be found at Arana Gulch, the Pogonip, Wilder Ranch, Schwan Lake, UCSC meadows, the San Lorenzo River, and any urban or suburban area.

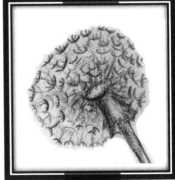

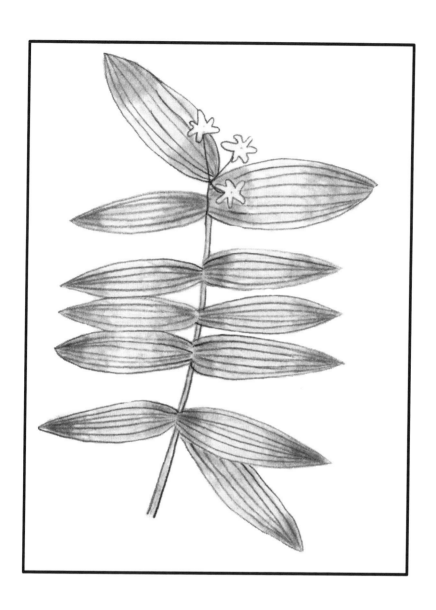

FALSE SOLOMON'S SEAL

Maianthemum stellatum,
Smilacina stellatum,
Maianthemum racemosum,
Smilacina racemosum

False Solomon's Seal is a low-growing perennial herb with a one to one and a half foot long stem. Protruding from the stem in a flat arrangement are shiny, dark green, pointed leaves with parallel veins. Blooming in May and June, False Solomon's Seal displays dainty, white, six-petaled flowers that surround the tip of the stem like miniature stars. The flowers then transform into clusters of vibrant, dark red berries. The berries are edible raw or cooked and are bittersweet in flavor.[1] Beneath ground-level, stringy roots branch form fibrous rhizomes. It is possible to eat these stringy rhizomes, but processing it in lye water and cooking is required. Many stems can connect to a single rhizome, creating condensed clusters of plants thriving on the forest floor.[2]

FALSE SOLOMON'S SEAL: NATURAL BAND-AID

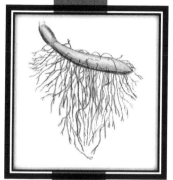

There are two main False Solomon's Seal species that grow in this region (*M. or S. racemosum* and *M. or S. stellata*), but they both serve the same medicinal purposes.[3]

EXTERNAL USAGE: False Solomon's Seal rhizomes can relieve cuts, bites, stings,[4] inflammations, poison oak rashes, boils, burns, gum irritations,[5] and swellings.[6]

INTERNAL USAGE: False Solomon's Seal rhizomes can be consumed for sore throats,[7] chest colds,[8] lung stability, and coughs, since False Solomon's Seal is an astringent.[9, 10]

PREPARATION: False Solomon's Seal's rhizomes can be applied externally to the skin as a poultice, salve, or survival band-aid made by slicing a cross section of the rhizome and applying to the inflicted area directly. For internal ailments, simply chewing on the fresh astringent rhizome can be sufficient. Additionally, False Solomon's Seal's fresh rhizomes can be prepared into a tincture, decoction, or cough syrup with honey. Dried rhizomes can also be handy to carry around for poultices and infusions in a first aid kit.[11]

WARNINGS: Because the rhizome only grows one-to-three inches every year, False Solomon's Seal is very vulnerable to overharvesting.[12]

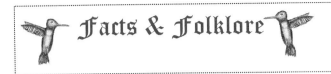

Facts & Folklore

The name "False Solomon's Seal" does this herb an injustice, for there is nothing false about it. This plant is just as useful as the "true" Solomon's Seal, and is not trying to imitate it.[13] False Solomon's Seal has been valued as a magical herb back to the time of Solomon, the third king of ancient Israel. The flowers of *M. racemosa* resemble the starry design on King Solomon's magical ring, which legends say he used to communicate with spirits and animals.[14] In North America, Native Americans mashed False Solomon's Seal's rhizomes and threw them into streams to stun fish.[15]

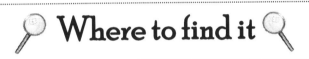

Where to find it

Habitats consisting of shady Redwood or California Bay forests with rich, damp soil will most likely host False Solomon's Seal. This herbaceous plant can be found on mountain slopes and near rivers or streams. I have identified this herb at Grey Whale Ranch, the Pogonip, Waddell Creek, and Henry Cowell.

To clarify, the genus *Smilacina* and the genus *Maianthemum* are considered exact synonyms, while the species *racemosum* and *stellatum* both proliferate throughout California.

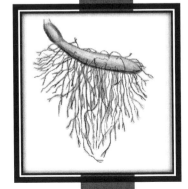

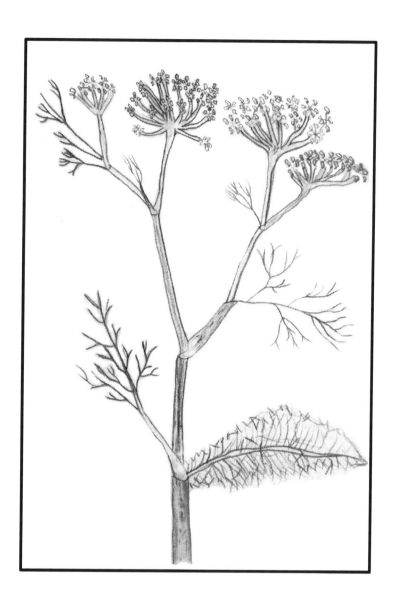

FENNEL

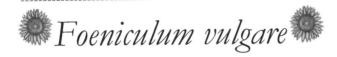

Foeniculum vulgare

Fennel is a three to five foot high perennial herb, with lacy tufts of needle-like leaves resembling billowy squirrel tails. All parts of Foeniculum vulgare *are edible and delicious, tasting sweet and spicy like licorice. Yellow oblong flowers grow in flat tufts atop the bushy plants, becoming grayish-brown seeds in autumn.*

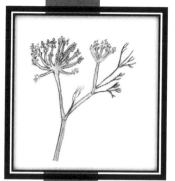

FENNEL: SOOTHING THE DIGESTIVE SYSTEM

INTERNAL USAGE: Fennel's main medicinal purpose is soothing the digestive system, since Fennel is a carminative[1] and anti-spasmodic.[2] By consuming the leaves, stem, root, and seeds, one may feel instantaneous relief from stomach discomforts such as indigestion, gas, cramps, colic, and irritable bowel syndrome.[3] Additionally, Fennel seeds are used to stimulate breast milk production, and soothe coughs and sore throats.[4] *Foeniculum vulgare* is a diuretic, diaphoretic, and anti-microbial.[5]

EXTERNAL USAGE: The seeds and leaf poultice will heal infected gums and toothaches when applied to the mouth directly.[6]

PREPARATION: The seeds can be prepared into an infusion, tincture, or syrup, while the entire plant can be consumed raw to release medicinal properties.[7]

WARNINGS: Don't use medicinally during pregnancy, since this plant can lead to miscarriage. Culinary use is fine in small amounts.[8] Although I don't see that much resemblance, Fennel can be mistaken for Poison Hemlock (*Conium maculatum*). Be sure to identify this plant properly, as the consequences are fatal if Poison Hemlock is injested.[9]

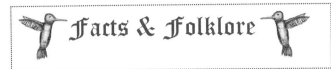

Facts & Folklore

The Egyptians, Chinese, Greeks, Hindus, Sumerians, and Anglo-Saxons have used Fennel medicinally and for culinary purposes for more than 5,000 years.[10] The Greek word for Fennel is "Marathon" after the battle of Marathon which took place in a field of Fennel in 490 B.C.[11] In tenth-century England, Fennel was one of the nine sacred herbs thought to heal every illness.[12] Fennel, native to the Mediterranean region of Europe, grows in Asia, Europe, and North America.[13]

 # Where to find it

When exploring Santa Cruz, one is bound to discover Fennel. This herb is copious in open regions such as meadows, fields, abandoned gardens, and forest edges. I have seen this wild edible in UCSC meadows, Grey Whale, Wilder Ranch, the Pogonip, meadows behind Blue Ball Park, the lower San Lorenzo River, and Harken Slough in Watsonville. Fennel also grows on roadsides such as Highway 1 and Highway 17, specifically at the Lexington Reservoir.

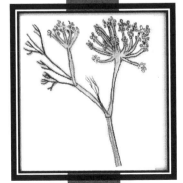

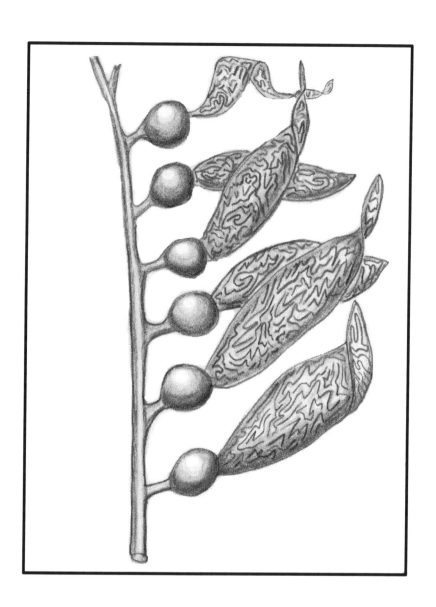

GIANT KELP

 Macrocystis pyrifera

Giant Kelp is a common brown seaweed with a long stem that often reaches lengths of more than one hundred and fifty feet. These sea plants' thick and tough stems are fun to play with at the beach. In the ocean, Giant Kelp can grow as much as two feet per day. Attached to the stalk are hollow, bulbous bladders filled with air that keep Giant Kelp floating towards the surface, enabling the entire plant to photosynthesize. Hanging off the bulbs are thick, leathery, ribbon-like leaves called blades. These brown blades have distinctive grooves in a complex, maze-like pattern. The blades, as well as the rest of the plant, contain a substance called algen, giving Giant Kelp a slimy, snot-like consistency. Giant Kelp is anchored to the ocean floor by a root system called a holdfast. Sea Otters anchor in the Giant Kelp by wrapping themselves in a floating raft of this seaweed.

GIANT KELP: SOOTHING THE RESPIRATORY SYSTEM AND RESTORING MINERAL BALANCE

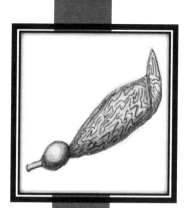

Macrocystis pyrifera is a species of brown sea algae, a category of seaweeds that have many useful healing properties. Although other species of brown sea algaes have been researched and used for thousands of years, Giant Kelp, which only grows along the coast from Baja to Alaska, is a newly studied species. Since Giant Kelp is directly related to other brown sea algaes, this seaweed presumably has similar uses, yet more research is needed to prove this individual species' effectiveness. Researchers are discovering more uses for Giant Kelp all the time.

INTERNAL USAGE: Brown sea algaes can soothe coughs, lungs, irritated throats, and are expectorant. Kelp is anti-inflammatory, which can soothe mucous membranes, ulcers, and heal tissue damage.[1] In addition, brown sea algaes can prove beneficial to sensory nerves, brain tissues, and the spinal cord. Brown sea algaes can also treat thyroid, prostate, and lymph node enlargements.[2]

All Kelp is extremely rich in iodine, which is beneficial, since many people are iodine deficient. In addition to iodine, brown sea algae contains antioxidants, proteins, and minerals such as potassium, iron, selenium, magnesium, phosphorus, sodium, zinc, and calcium.[3] Brown sea algae also supplies the body with vitamins such as A, C, D, E, K and numerous B vitamins.[4] The iodine in Kelp, along with the other vitamins and minerals, help with hair loss, effects of radiation, obesity, mental illnesses, thyroid gland problems, and replenishment and moisturizing of the skin.[5]

PREPARATION: For information on preparing Giant Kelp, see "Harvesting and Preparing Giant Kelp" in "Recipes."

WARNINGS: Giant Kelp should not be consumed by people with deficient stomachs and spleens,[6] and those who are iodine-sensitive.[7] Overconsumption of Giant Kelp may lead to thyroid imbalances and reactions from too much iodine.[8]

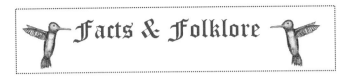

Facts & Folklore

Kelp has been regarded very highly in parts of Asia such as China and Japan. In Japan, Kelp and other seaweeds are referred to as "Heaven Grass." In China, Kelps were offered as sacrificial food for the gods.[9] All Kelps are edible and have great nutritional benefits. Kelp and other sea vegetables have been an important part of the diet in Asia for thousands of years.[10]

 # Where to find it

Giant Kelp grows in whole forests throughout the entire waters of the Monterey Bay, as well as most spots north along the Pacific Ocean. Since Giant Kelp is the main sea plant in Santa Cruz, this herb is one of the easiest to identify and find. Manresa, Rio Del Mar, and coves off West Cliff are examples of ideal places for harvesting. Giant Kelp may contain heavy metals like cadmium, mercury, lead, and arsenic, due to seawater pollution, so do not collect Giant Kelp in areas where those metals are known to occur in high quantities.[11] Check the water quality online for your given spot before harvesting. (See "Harvesting and Preparing Giant Kelp" in "Recipes.")

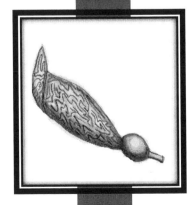

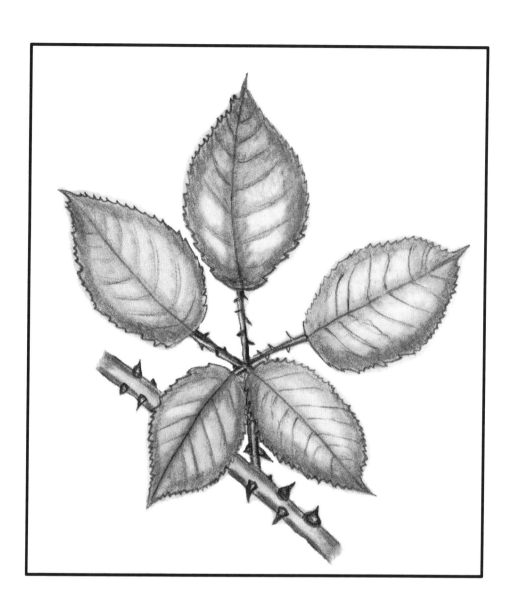

HIMALAYAN BLACKBERRY

 Rubus armeniacus

Himalayan Blackberry is an invasive vine that grows in four-to-six-foot high dense thickets, completely covering the area of growth. Surrounding the thick stalks are large, painfully sharp thorns. Normally growing in groups of five, Himalayan Blackberry leaves are oval shaped, serrated, and hairy, with small thorns on the underside of each leaf. White, five-petaled flowers ripen into delicious, sweet blackberries that contain a dark red juice. Made up of tiny subdivisions called drupelets, these berries fruit in late June and July, an exciting part of every summer. Himalayan Blackberry differs from the native variety, which have very small thorns and produce tart berries in the early spring.

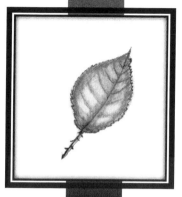

HIMALAYAN BLACKBERRY: ASTRINGENT FOR THE MOUTH, SKIN, AND DIGESTIVE TRACT

Rubus armeniacus not only produces delicious, nutritious blackberries, but has astringent properties as well.

EXTERNAL USAGE: Externally, Himalayan Blackberry's astringent properties are useful as an acne treatment for oily and large pored skin.[1] (See "Himalayan Blackberry Astringent" in "Recipes.") In addition, Himalayan Blackberry's astringent qualities can soothe mouth ulcers, sore throats, thrush, and inflamed gums when used as a mouthwash.[2] The leaves can help skin afflictions, as this herb can minimize bleeding.[3]

INTERNAL USAGE: Internally, Himalayan Blackberry's astringent tannins help cure diarrhea, dysentery,[4] hemorrhoids,[5] and cholera.[6] *Rubus armeniacus* is a diuretic and depurative and may also assist with anemia, regulating menstruation, gout, and bleeding gums.[7] Himalayan Blackberry can be made into a delicious cough syrup for colds,[8] sore throats,[9] and expectorant properties.[10]

PREPARATION: The roots, leaves, and young stalks, preferably fresh, should be made into an infusion or tincture in order for the astringent properties to be released.[11] One can also make a syrup from the berries and roots.[12] Externally, the infusion can be used as a mouthwash or skin rinse, or the fresh leaves can be used as a poultice.[13]

WARNINGS: No known cautions.

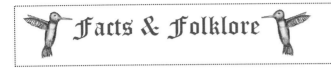

Facts & Folklore

Himalayan Blackberry originated in Armenia and Iran and was introduced to Europe, North America, and Australia in the 1800's. Himalayan Blackberry is now naturalized throughout most of the world and considered an invasive species.[14] Since Himalayan Blackberry contains vitamin C, the settlers who came to California ate blackberries regularly as a cure for scurvy, a terrible disease caused by vitamin C deficiency.[15] The berries are an excellent source of B vitamins such as B2 and B6, fiber, manganese, antioxidants, and ellagic, pantothenic, and folic acids.[16] Himalayan Blackberry has been employed to keep animals out of villages, due to the sharp thorns.[17] The fibers of the stem were used by Native Americans as strong cordage. The berry juices make an excellent bluish-purple dye.[18]

 # Where to find it

Since Himalayan Blackberry is extremely invasive, it grows EVERYWHERE! Blackberry is common on roadsides, meadows, suburban sites, abandoned gardens, and every other open ecosystem. Himalayan Blackberry can grow in a wide range of different soils.[19] I have found Himalayan Blackberry at Waddell Creek, the Pogonip, Arana Gulch, Henry Cowell, Schwan Lake, Neary Lagoon, Natural Bridges, and the Market Street Canal. Himalayan Blackberry and Poison Oak are often found growing together, since they share similar habitats, so look carefully before you harvest this plant!

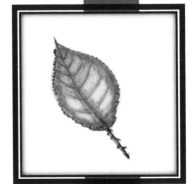

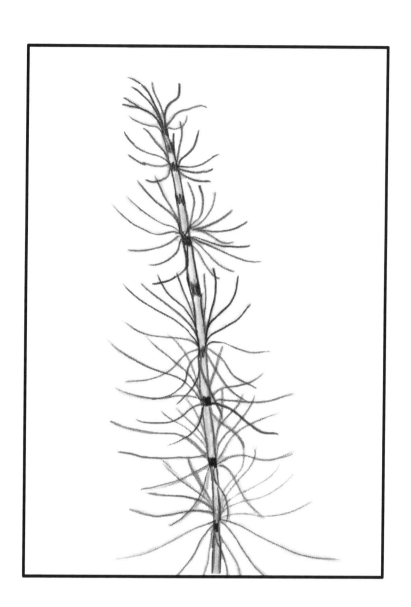

HORSETAIL

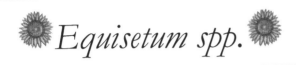

Equisetum spp.

Horsetail, a unique prehistoric plant, is a straight, one-to-four foot high river reed. Equisetum *has many rings of skinny needles protruding from the stalk, resembling a horse's tail. The stalk is stacked with one-to-three inch segments, similar to bamboo. Horsetail reproduces by rhizomes, and sends spores to float in the wind, just little packets of DNA without any guarantee of their survival.*

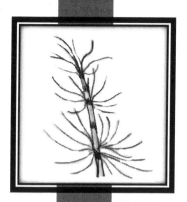

HORSETAIL: CURING THE BLADDER AND KIDNEYS

INTERNAL USAGE: Horsetail can heal bladder infections and general kidney issues such as kidney stones.[1] Horsetail can also be used for withdrawing fluid buildup in the legs. Some *Equisetum* species are classified as diuretics.[2] Additionally, Horsetail can be employed to stop bleeding in the respiratory system, nose, or stomach.[3] Horsetail contains silica, calcium, and other minerals, which strengthen bones, hair, and fingernails, since those body parts require high mineral levels.[4] Horsetail decoction can be consumed for up to a month to heal broken bones.[5]

EXTERNAL USAGE: Horsetail is an antimicrobial and anti-inflammatory to the skin, which can draw the pus out of boils and sores.[6]

PREPARATION: A tincture, decoction, vinegar,[7] compress, poultice, powder extract[8] or salve can be made from the fresh, aerial parts.[9] The decoction or tincture can be taken internally.[10] Externally, all *Equisetum* species can be made into an effective poison oak rinse with vinegar. (See "Poison Oak Rinse" in "Recipes".)

WARNINGS: *Equisetum* is not a heavily researched herb, so the internal uses may have unknown side effects.[11] Use during pregnancy is not recommended, although there is no proof of any harm.[12] This herb is known to break down the vitamin thiamine when injested, possibly not leaving enough in the body.[13] In addition, consuming Horsetail might decrease potassium levels in the body.[14] It is best to stay on the safe side if you are vitamin deficient until further research is announced.

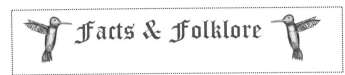

Facts & Folklore

Equisetum is the only living species in the class *Equisetopsida*, which thrived for over 100 million years in the forests of the late Paleozoic age. Some *Equisetopsida*, like Calamites, grew to 100 feet high![15] Fossils of Calamite trunks have been uncovered from 310 million years ago, proving that the unique looking horsetails of today are living representations of how life looked long ago.[16] Equisetum has a rough surface due to its high silica quantity, so this plant has been used by Europeans and Native Americans as a sandpaper to scour cooking materials and to sand and file objects.[17]

 # Where to find it

When one is near any riverbed or location with damp soil, Horsetails will likely be found in large and dense clusters, resembling a miniature prehistoric forest. I have harvested this plant along the San Lorenzo River and have spotted this river reed at Waddell Creek and Ano Nuevo areas, Graham Hill Road, Grey Whale Ranch, across the road from Natural Bridges, and in shady, wet areas of UCSC close to the Arboretum. A common ornamental *Equisetum* species with clumps of tall bare stalks is often grown for its unique appearance, and is cultivated in various public landscapings, including the Santa Cruz Yacht Harbor.

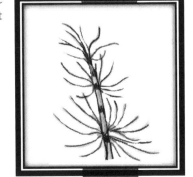

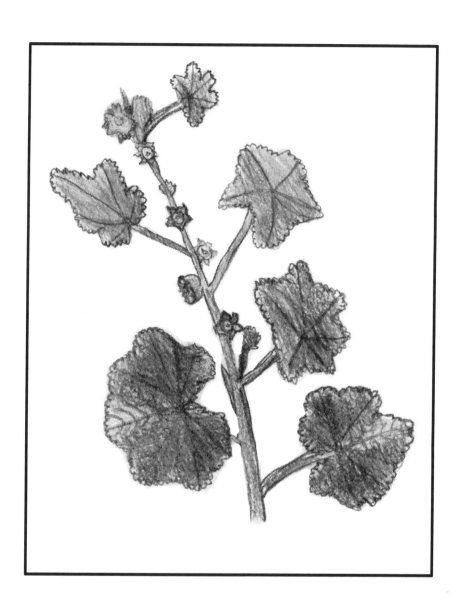

MALLOW

Malva parviflora
Malva neglecta

*Mallows (*Malva *species) are common weeds that grow from six inches to three feet high in California. Mallows have five rounded lobes on each serrated leaf. The leaves and round seeds are edible and nutritious, although not with any exuberant flavor.[1] Mallows contain a substance called mucilage in every part of the plant, giving this herb a slimy, wet consistency that you can taste and feel. The flowers are white to light pink or purple. The species* M. parviflora *and* M. neglecta *are often referred to as Cheeseweed because the seed-heads resemble cheese rounds, with each individual seed in a wedge shape.[2]*

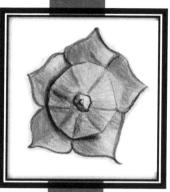

MALLOW: SLIMY, SOOTHING HEALER

INTERNAL USAGE: Due to Mallow's mucilaginous nature, this weed can soothe the body. The slimy mucilage can line and comfort the digestive, urinary, and respiratory tracts, and treat coughs, colds, and influenza.[3] Mallow can prevent kidney inflammation and kidney stones and may prove an excellent immune booster. Mallow can additionally be used as a shampoo, hair softener, and treatment for dandruff.[4]

EXTERNAL USAGE: Externally, Mallow can heal swelling, sores, and boils, and replenish the skin.[5]

PREPARATION: An infusion of the fresh leaves and a decoction or tincture of the fresh roots should be manufactured for this plant's internal medicinal qualities. Fresh Mallow roots make an excellent addition to cough tincture recipes. Externally, a fresh leaf poultice should be prepared.[6]

WARNINGS: Use caution when harvesting Malvas in nitrogen-rich soils because the leaves can contain high nitrate levels, especially in croplands.[7]

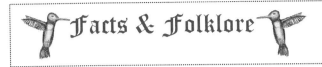

Facts & Folklore

Malva comes from the Greek word *malakos*, which means soft, describing the slimy energetic.[8] Before gelatin was used in marshmallows, industries prepared the slimy roots of Malva's relative, Marsh Mallow (*Althea officinalis*), to create this concession.[9] Mallows originated in the Mediterranean and southern European regions, but have naturalized throughout the world.[10] Since Mallows are nutritious weeds, they have been consumed throughout history for survival in wartime or crop failure.[11] Mallow leaves are a great addition to salads or stir-fries; when consumed they can act as an immune booster and supply nutrition.[12] Mallow leaves contain iron, manganese, potassium, selenium, copper, zinc, phosphorous, and magnesium,[13] while the entire plant contains large quantities of minerals, vitamins A and C, and protein.[14] Native Americans used Mallow for its medicinal uses,[15] while in Egypt, Mallow is still cultivated as an essential food crop.[16] I enjoy wildcrafting the woody, stringy stems into strong cordage.

Where to find it

Mallows flourish in open areas such as gardens, meadows, fields, roadsides, wastelands, and cropland habitats. Mallow can be found at Arana Gulch, UCSC meadows, the Pogonip, Wilder Ranch, and Waddel Creek. Wild Geranium can look similar to Mallow, and share the same habitat. However, Wild Geranium seeds are long and skinny, while Mallow seeds are small and round.

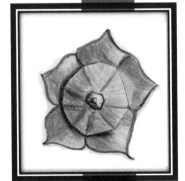

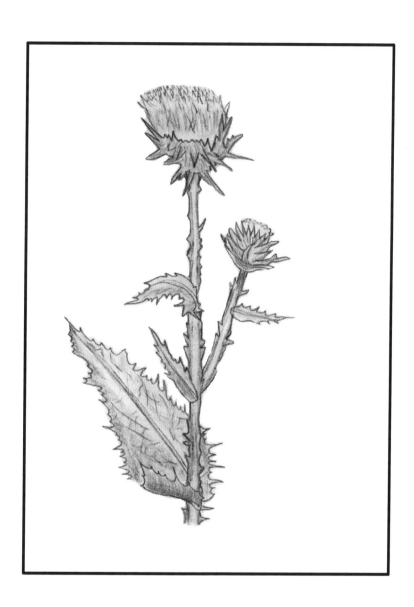

MILK THISTLE

 Silybum marianum

Milk Thistle is a bulky, herbaceous weed that generally grows from three to five feet in height. The entire plant is extremely prickly since the edges of the leaves and flower heads are covered in sharp, painful spines, causing most people to avoid this weed. However, if the spines are removed, the leaves are delicious, and the thinner stems are juicy and sweet. The stems, leaves, and flower heads are all edible raw or boiled. Milk Thistle has an enchanting white, web-like pattern on the surface of each wide, green, foot long leaf. On top of each tall stem lies a flower head which produces a bright purple flower. Sticking out horizontally from the large flower head are long, needle like spines. In summer, the flower heads burst into seed, releasing white fluff meant to carry the black seeds away. Silybum marianum *grows from winter until midsummer.*

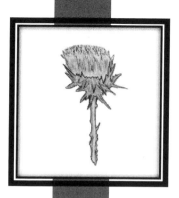

MILK THISTLE: CURING LIVER DISORDERS

INTERNAL USAGE: Although Milk Thistle is disguised as a prickly weed, this herb has powerful liver-relieving powers. Milk Thistle cures liver disorders, including damage caused by chemicals, too much alcohol, poison, chronic hepatitis, jaundice, and chronic liver inflammation.[1] Milk Thistle is the only substance capable of preventing Deathcap Mushroom's deadly effects on the liver.[2] Other uses of Milk Thistle include healing gallbladder complaints, kidney damage, spleen diseases, lung inflammation, prostate cancer, and benign prostatic hyperplasia. In addition, Milk Thistle has been known to lower high cholesterol by decreasing inflammation of the heart, a cause of heart disease.[3]

EXTERNAL USAGE: Externally, the above-ground parts can be applied to the skin in the event of toxicity from too much radiation.[4]

PREPARATION: *Silybum marianum's* seeds are most commonly used in a preparation, mostly as a tincture. The above-ground parts, such as the leaves, can be consumed through the digestive tract or tinctured along with the seeds.[5]

WARNINGS: Do not take Milk Thistle during pregnancy, with certain medical conditions, or while taking prescription drugs.[6]

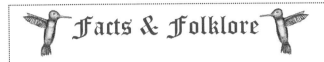

Facts & Folklore

Milk Thistle is a nutritious food and has been consumed throughout history as a vegetable. Milk Thistle is commonly eaten in Mediterranean countries, specifically in rural areas.[7] The artichoke is the most famous member of the Thistle family, although Milk Thistle is just as nourishing.[8] Milk Thistle has been thought of as an herb of protection. Milk Thistle has been known to give strength and energy, ensure protection against evils, and call spirits.[9]

 # Where to find it

Milk Thistle will plant itself in any open or partially shaded area such as a meadow, forest edge, or roadside, usually in dense patches. I have enjoyed getting to know this tough weed at the Santa Cruz Yacht Harbor near the Lighthouse, Arana Gulch, San Lorenzo Park, Ocean View Park, Harkins Slough in Watsonville, and Wilder Ranch.

Italian Thistle (*Carduus pycnocephalus*) is another Thistle common in Santa Cruz County. Although edible, this small, skinny species is not proven to be effective for medicine in the same way as Milk Thistle.

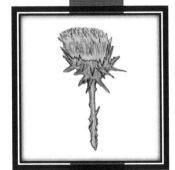

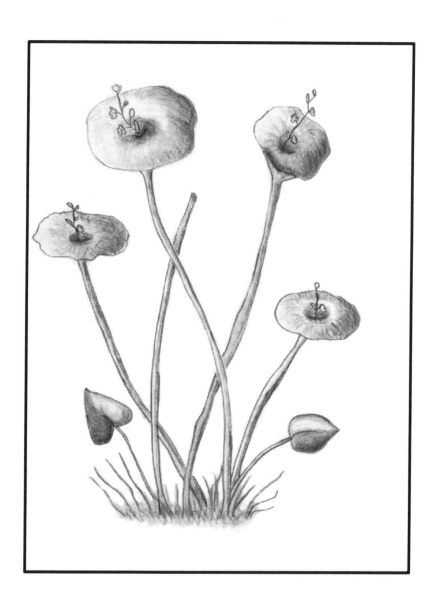

MINER'S LETTUCE

 Claytonia perfoliata (subsp. mexicana)

Miner's Lettuce is a dainty, low-growing annual herb that pops up every winter. Claytonia perfoliata (subsp. mexicana) *either consists of heart-shaped, low-growing, small leaves, or broad, circular leaves that look like miniature umbrellas resting atop thick, juicy stems. The stems contain a stringy fiber at the center, ideal for cordage or emergency thread. On top of the circular leaves lie cute, tiny white or pink flowers. Miner's Lettuce is edible and delicious, tasting similar to spinach, but much juicier. This water-filled plant may possess a bulb, or just have a fibrous root system. Miner's Lettuce exists until late spring or early summer, when it drops its seeds and wilts away.*

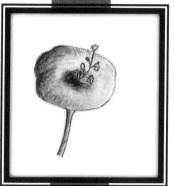

MINER'S LETTUCE: RESTORING NUTRITIOUS BALANCE AND PURIFYING THE BODY

INTERNAL USAGE: Miner's Lettuce is high in vitamins and minerals, including vitamin C, vitamin A, and iron.[1] Miner's Lettuce works especially well in combination with Stinging Nettle to restore the body to nutritious balance.[2] The high vitamin C content will prevent scurvy and can benefit the immune system.[3] Miner's Lettuce can be purifying and support the lymph and blood.[4] Additionally, Miner's Lettuce can act as an excellent detoxifier, disposing of heavy metals and toxins contained in the liver. This is due to nutrients rich in anti-oxidants, such as vitamin C, as well as chlorophyll.[5]

Miner's Lettuce, also called Winter Parslane,[6] is presumed to contain high quantities of Omega-3 fatty acids,[7] since this herb is in the Parslane family, *Portulacca*.[8] Omega-3 fatty acids have anti-inflammatory actions, specifically counteracting the inflammatory effects of Omega-6 fats, which are common in many foods.[9] Furthermore, *Claytonia perfoliata* can act as a mild laxative and effective diuretic.[10]

EXTERNAL USAGE: This spring vegetable can be made into a poultice of the mashed plant for rheumatic joints to relieve pain.[11]

PREPARATION: The nutritious and medicinal advantages can be released into the body by simply snacking on the juicy leaves and stems of *Claytonia perfoliata*.

WARNINGS: No known cautions.

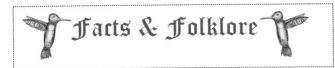

Facts & Folklore

The common name Miner's Lettuce originated from its use in the California Gold Rush. The miners ate significant amounts of this juicy plant to get their vitamin C intake, preventing scurvy.[12] Miner's Lettuce was brought from North America to Europe, where it was admired for its high quantity of vitamin C, and naturalized rapidly, becoming a common weed in places like England.[13] Native Americans ate *Claytonia perfoliata* as part of their diet. They put this plant on the trails of ants, so that acid from the ants would rub off on the leaves and flavor them.[14]

 # Where to find it

Every winter and spring, Miner's Lettuce thrives in cool, damp habitats under trees. It grows in forests, shady mountain slopes, and under oak trees. This juicy plant can be found in locations such as the Pogonip, Arboretum, Wilder Ranch, Santa Cruz Yacht Harbor, and Henry Cowell.

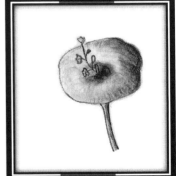

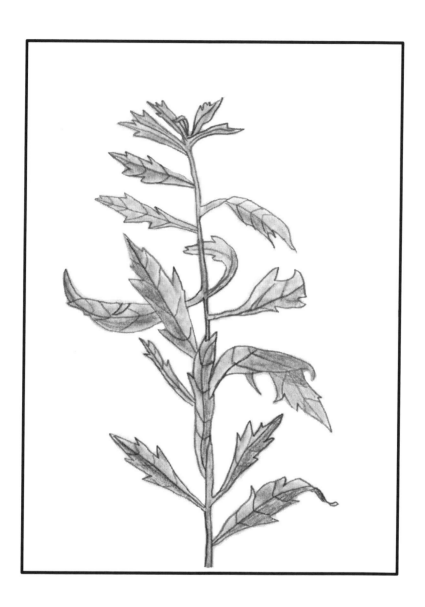

MUGWORT

 Artemisia douglasiana

Mugwort is a two to four foot high herbaceous plant with jagged, serrated leaves that grow densely upon a skinny, green or brown stem. The leaves that grow close to the top, especially on flowering stalks, tend to be almond-shaped and pointed, yet most Mugwort leaves are jagged and asymmetrical. Although green on top, the leaves are white on the underside. Artemisia douglasiana *gives off a spicy aroma, but tastes extremely bitter. Tiny, yellow flowers form in clusters towards the top foot or so of the stem. In late summer or autumn, the leaves and flowers dry on the brown stems but the plant still stands tall. Mugwort plants tend to grow close together, forming clusters.*

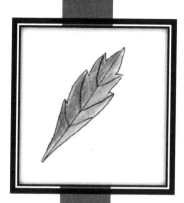

MUGWORT: RIDDING THE DIGESTIVE TRACT AND RELIEVING INFLAMMATION

INTERNAL USAGE: *Artemisia douglasiana* is a stomatic and antispasmodic, benefitting the digestive system by helping rid the body of gas, stomach acid, bloating, distension, worms, other parasites,[1] and diarrhea.[2] Mugwort can also stimulate the appetite. Mugwort's emenogogue, hemostatic, and antispasmodic qualities may assist with menstrual cramps,[3] some menopausal symptoms,[4] and heavy, extended menstrual flow.[5] Additionally, Mugwort is a nervine,[6] soothing the nerves[7] and mind, and relieving stress, insomnia, and anxiety.[8] Mugwort is a diaphoretic, reducing headaches and fevers.[9]

EXTERNAL USAGE: Externally, Mugwort leaves are anti-inflammatory, perfect for relieving Poison Oak.[10] (See "Poison Oak Rinse" in "Recipes.") Additionally, Mugwort is an anti-inflammatory, anti-microbial, and anesthetic, and may help heal sprains, bruises, and hyperextensions.[11]

PREPARATION: Mugwort leaves, flowers, and stems should be dried and prepared into an infusion[12] or tincture,[13] while the roots should be manufactured into a decoction or tincture.[14] For this herb's external preparations, the flowers in particular can be prepared into a salve, while the leaves can be placed into a poultice, infusion, or vinegar.[15]

WARNINGS: Consumption during pregnancy or breast feeding is strongly discouraged,[16] since Mugwort can stimulate the uterine lining.[17]

Facts & Folklore

In many Californian Native American languages, Mugwort means "dream herb." Mugwort is commonly believed to react with dreams: improving them, making recollection easier, and providing an enlightening and sacred sleep.[18] Mugwort has been burned as incense to ward away evil spirits, and dried for dream pillows to ward away wicked dreams.[19]

Mugwort has been in use for thousands of years in Traditional Chinese Medicine and Acupuncture in a process called Moxa, or Moxibustion.[20] This process involves the tip of a dried Mugwort stem to be ignited and held close to an area of the skin, generating heat and benefitting those with a cold or sluggish body type or ailment.[21] Moxa is also known to benefit the blood and maintain general health[22] by encouraging the flow of Qi, or life-force, believed by Traditional Chinese Medicine to run through certain channels of the body.[23] Applying Moxa directly to the skin or sticking a piece of burning Mugwort atop a needle is practiced in the burning of planter's warts.[24] Dried Mugwort leaves ignite very easily, which is why I enjoy using them for tinder to get fires burning quickly.

The name Artemisia originates from Artemis, the Greek Goddess of the hunt and the wild.[25]

 # Where to find it

Artemisia douglasiana grows in open or partially shady habitats, especially on riverbanks and forest edges. Mugwort exists plentifully at Henry Cowell, Rancho Del Oso, Old San Jose Road region, Wilder Ranch, the Bonny Doon Ecological Reserve, the Pogonip, and along the San Lorenzo River.

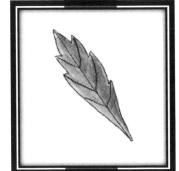

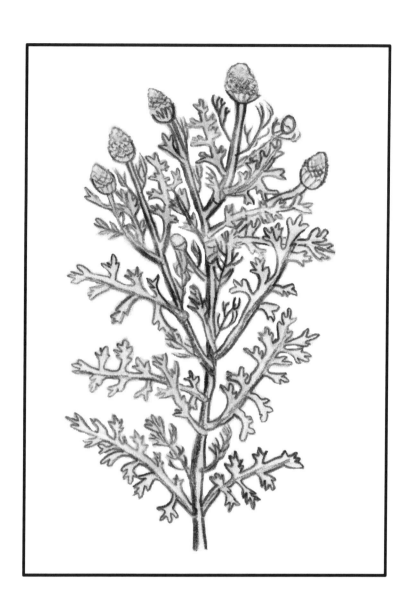

PINEAPPLE WEED

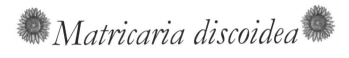

Matricaria discoidea

Pineapple Weed lives very close to the ground, never existing more than six inches in height. Pineapple Weeds possess fractal, yellow, petal-less flowers and lacy, branched, and pointed leaves. Matricaria discoidea's *cone shaped flowers have a scent and flavor of chamomile, since this herb is in same family. The smell has a sweet hint of pineapple, for which Pineapple Weed is named. After this annual sprouts in winter, stiff stems branch outwards and flowers form around April. This herb continues to thrive until September. Pineapple Weeds are edible and delicious, and fun to nibble on trails.*

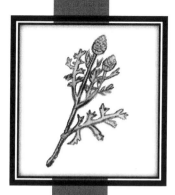

PINEAPPLE WEED: RELAXING THE DIGESTIVE SYSTEM

Pineapple Weed is equipped with sedative, antispasmodic, carminative, analgesic,[1] and antihemorrhagic properties.[2]

INTERNAL USAGE: *Matricaria discoidea* is beneficial towards the digestive system, and can treat upset stomachs, diarrhea, indigestion,[3] intestinal worms,[4] irritable bowel syndrome, stomach ulcers, and gas.[5] Pineapple Weed's mild sedative effects can also soothe contractions of the stomach muscles[6] and help with insomnia and anxiety.[7] Pineapple Weed has been consumed by women for relief from menstrual cramps[8] and pains[9] and to encourage milk production.[10] In addition, *Matricaria discoidea* might reduce colds, fevers,[11] and influenza.[12]

EXTERNAL USAGE: Externally, Pineapple Weed's flowers can be employed to heal wounds, leg ulcers, burns, sunburn,[13] itching,[14] and infected sores.[15]

PREPARATION: A handful of Pineapple Weed's fresh or dried[16] young flower heads can be steeped in an herbal infusion, which tastes similar to Chamomile, yet is sweeter.[17] The leaves can also be used, although they add a bitter flavor.[18] A tincture is also a possible internal preparation, although the infusion is mild, pleasant, and easy to prepare.[19] Pineapple Weed's external properties will be released as a bath, soak, or poultice.[20]

WARNINGS: If you have seasonal allergies, be aware that Pineapple Weed may cause allergic reactions.[21] Experiment hesitantly, until you are sure that this wonderful herb will not aggravate your system.

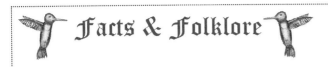

Facts & Folklore

Pineapple weed was most likely native to Northeastern Asia initially, yet spread to Europe in the 1800's when it was introduced to North America.[22] Kootenai Indian tribes once used the whole plant to keep any insects away from food.[23] Pineapple Weed has also been used by Native Americans as a sweetly scented pillow stuffer and a perfume for the skin.[24] Additionally, Native tribes strung the flower heads as beads.[25] Since Pineapple Weed has been known to repel insects, an infusion prepared from the dried flowers can be splashed on the skin in order to be insect-free.[26] The flower heads can be added to stir-fries, casseroles, salads, and many more recipes.[27]

 # Where to find it

Pineapple Weed prefers soil that is rocky, compacted, and poor, where humans have disturbed the earth with vehicles, pedestrian paths, and roads.[28] Pineapple Weed also requires locations where there is limited competition from other weeds and grasses.[29] One can find Pineapple Weed defining the sides of paths in meadows, suburban areas, in sidewalk cracks, and throughout disturbed ground. Sprouting during winter or early spring, Pineapple Weed lives in Arana Gulch, UCSC meadows, Grey Whale, the Pogonip, and Wilder Ranch. In addition, Pineapple Weed grows at Lighthouse Field, where I have early memories of nibbling flower heads while exploring the meadows there. Make sure to harvest this plant in dog-free zones, or at least use caution.

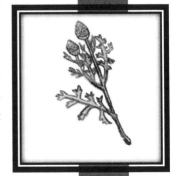

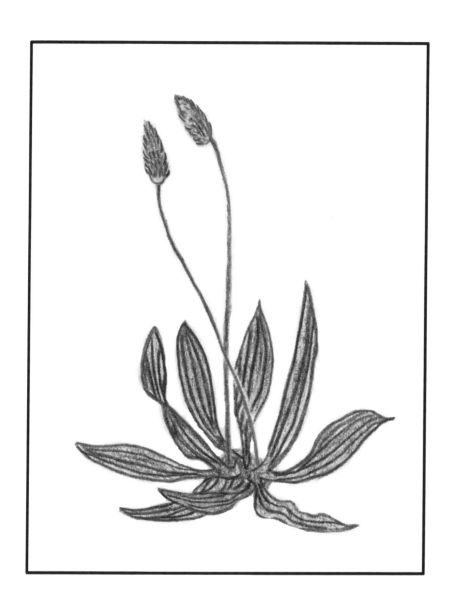

PLANTAIN

Plantago lanceolata

Plantain is a perennial herb that grows to one and a half feet high, with a cluster of long, narrow, pointed, parallel-veined leaves that jet out from the base. The leaves are edible, although not particularly palatable in excessive amounts, due to this plant's astringent nature. In winter, corn-like, intricate seed heads rise a foot above the leaf cluster atop skinny stems. At first, miniature white flowers reach out from the green heads, but then the heads turn brown, fuzzy, and dry, and seeds form. Plantain tops are edible, and can be eaten raw, roasted, in dishes,[1] or in a mush with hot water. Plantain contains high quantities of calcium and vitamins A and C.[2]

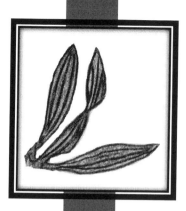

PLANTAIN: EXTRACTING MATERIAL FROM WOUNDS

EXTERNAL USAGE: *Plantago lanceolata* has amazing external healing properties, due to its astringent, anti-inflammatory, and anti-bacterial qualities.[3] Plantain can heal wounds such as burns, scrapes, cuts, infections,[4] rashes, eczema,[5] and boils.[6] I have been personally impressed with Plantain's ability to extract foreign substances from wounds, since Plantain can draw out splinters and venom and can heal bug bites and stings.[7]

INTERNAL USAGE: Plantain may relieve respiratory tract inflammations, including bronchitis, colds, and dry coughs.[8] Furthermore, Plantain can treat gastrointestinal problems such as diarrhea,[9] ulcers,[10] and dysentery.[11] Urinary tract inflammations such as cystitis[12] may be cured by Plantain due to diuretic and astringent effects.[13] Lastly, Plantain can release internal anti-bacterial effects to the body.[14]

PREPARATION: A salve, poultice, infusion, syrup, or tincture can be made from the fresh leaves.[15] (See "All Purpose Salve" in "Recipes.") The internal anti-bacterial effects cannot be relied upon when heated, so a tincture or syrup from the fresh leaf juice is recommended.[16] *P. major* and *P. lanceolata* are both used in medicine and possess the same medicinal uses.[17]

WARNINGS: No cautions known.

Facts & Folklore

Plantain has been recognized throughout history as a medicinal herb. *Plantago lanceolata* and *Plantago major* both originated in Asia and Europe,[18] and were brought over by the British to the Americas.[19] According to legend, Alexander the Great (356 BC – 323 BC) found Plantain and brought it back with him to Europe,[20] using the herb to cure his headaches.[21] Native Americans, who were already accomplished in the studying of herbs, were introduced to plantain by settlers, and some tribes used this plant for external purposes.[22] Native Americans referred to Plantain as "white man's footsteps" since this weed seemed to spring up everywhere that the settlers journeyed.[23, 24]

The Anglo-Saxons believed Plantain to have extraordinary healing properties, listing the herb as one of nine sacred plants. Ancient Persians and Arabians incorporated Plantain for its digestive system uses.[25]

 # Where to find it

Plantain lives in most open areas of Santa Cruz, thriving in meadows, fields, gardens, roadsides, and suburban regions. Plantain flourishes at Arana Gulch, the Arboretum, the Pogonip, UCSC meadows, Wilder Ranch, and the meadows behind Blue Ball Park. *Plantago major*, or Broadleaf Plantain, also exists in this region, but only in mowed, grassy lawns at parks, where I wouldn't recommend harvesting due to herbicide spray. Harvesting *Plantago lanceolata*, or the Narrowleaf Plantain variety that occurs wild in Santa Cruz, is certainly the best option.

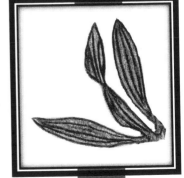

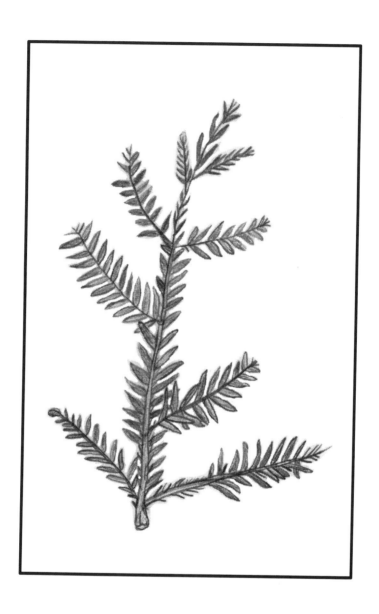

REDWOOD

 Sequoia sempervirens

Redwood is a world-famous tree, known for its astonishing size and majestic height; it is the tallest tree in the world, often reaching heights of over 300 feet.[1] The bark is spongy, soft, thick, and reddish brown in color, giving Redwood its name. The needles are clusters of many short, evergreen needles, skinny and pointed in shape. The leaves become a golden brown color when they die and fall, creating an enchanting forest floor of decomposing debris. Sequoia sempervirens reproduce by intricate seed pods that require fire to open, but can also reproduce by shooting saplings from the root system. Redwood trees acquire more than half of their moisture from fog, which is why they thrive in coastal California.[2] Redwood trees are very familiar to me, since I have grown up experiencing the beauty of these wise and ancient wonders, for which I am forever grateful.

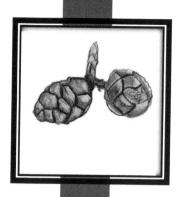

REDWOOD:
EASING THE LUNGS
AND THROAT

Sequoia sempervirens contains a rich, powerful medicine that enhances the majestic grandeur of this ancient tree.

INTERNAL USAGE: Redwood is an expectorant, antimicrobial, and aromatic herb, ideal for clearing mucus congestion in the lungs[3] and opening the breathing pathways.[4] *Sequoia sempervirens* can cure chest colds,[5] head colds, and influenza.[6] When Redwood infusion is consumed, the antimicrobial aromatic oils travel through the bloodstream and out of the lungs, fighting infections along the way.[7] Additionally, Redwood's aromatic and astringent properties can soothe the urinary tract and ease mild bladder infections.[8] Redwood needles have high concentrations of vitamin C, benefitting the immune system and preventing scurvy, a terrible disease caused by vitamin C deficiency.[9] Lastly, Redwood is a circulatory stimulant[10] and relaxes the muscles and nervous system.[11]

EXTERNAL USAGE: Native American tribes such as the Kashaya Pomo people made a poultice out of Redwood foliage for the treatment of earaches.[12]

PREPARATION: Dried Redwood needles should be prepared into an infusion, steam inhalation,[13] or tincture for its internal properties to be released. Trim off a branch of fresh Redwood needles and hang upside down for at least three weeks until fully dry; surprisingly, the fresh needles do not infuse as well as the dried. (See "Redwood Infusion" in "Recipes.")

WARNINGS: No cautions known.

Facts & Folklore

In the 1800's, the fate of these beautiful native trees devastatingly changed. When American settlers journeyed westward to California, they wanted wood to satisfy their ambitious needs.[14] As more people colonized and the Gold Rush began, commercial logging of *Sequoia sempervirens* and *gigantea* (which covered most of California at that time) expanded drastically. Redwoods decreased even more rapidly as the industry became more complex, with large scale logging and trains for wood transportation. By the 1990's, **95 percent of the original forests have been cleared!** [15]

Prior to the 1800's, the native peoples of this region lived with these trees for thousands of years, and adapted well to this ecosystem.[16] This herbaceous tree was sacred to specific tribes, who believed that bad luck came to those who cut them down. They even tried to persuade the new Americans not to cut down these mighty trees, to no avail.[17]

 # Where to find it

The only region in the world that *Sequoia sempervirens* grows is along a thin strip on the California coast from around the Oregon border to southern Monterey County.[18] The location in Santa Cruz that I know best is Henry Cowell State Park, a vast Redwood grove near Felton. In addition, more Redwood hotspots include Big Basin, Little Basin, Felton and Boulder Creek regions, Fall Creek, Grey Whale Ranch, UCSC, Rancho Del Oso, Old San Jose Road, Nisene Marks, and along many roads and freeways such as Highway 17.

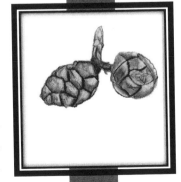

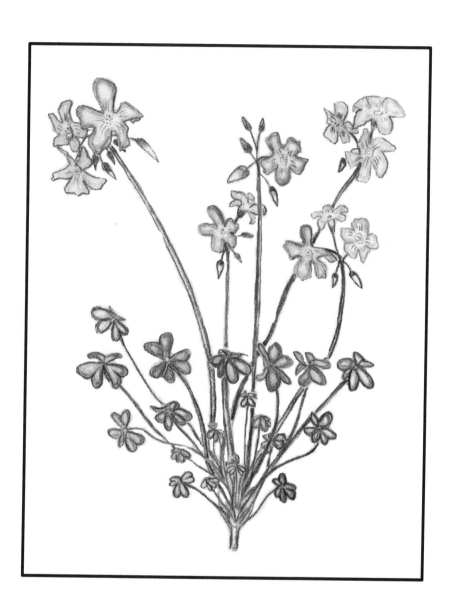

SOUR GRASS

Oxalis pes-caprae

From a very young age, I loved snacking on Sour Grass, one of my first plant connections. Sour Grass is a common name for Oxalis pes-caprae, a species in the Oxalis genus, which takes up the great majority of the Wood Sorrel family, Oxalidaceae.[1] Wood Sorrels can be identified by sets of three heart-shaped leaflets that lie on the tip of each short, skinny stem. These leaves are dark green on top, but greenish-white on the underside. Oxalis pes-caprae's flower stems can grow over one-and-a-half feet high and are stringy and juicy. Resting atop these stems are bright yellow, five petaled, cheery flowers and many cone-shaped buds. Orange stamens nest in the center of each inch-wide flower.

Sour Grass is edible and very sour to the taste, but in a delicious, non-bitter way.[2] This sour flavor results from a compound called oxalic acid, contained inside the stems, leaves, and flowers. Although they also contain the component oxalic acid, Docks and Sorrels are classified in the Buckwheat family, Polygonaceae.[3]

Oxalis pes-caprae should not be confused with Oxalis stricta, another Oxalis with yellow flowers that also lives in Santa Cruz. In order to limit confusion, notice that Oxalis pes-caprae is tall and has a vertical root with bulbs attached. In contrast, Oxalis stricta, along many other Oxalis varieties, are smaller with far-branching roots and skinny seed pods, which burst open to scatter the seeds.[4] All plants in the Oxalis genus have similar uses.[5]

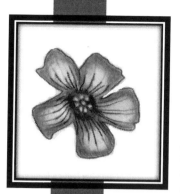

SOUR GRASS: HEALING THE DIGESTIVE SYSTEM AND STAUNCHING BLOOD

INTERNAL USAGE: Plants in the Wood Sorrel family, including *Oxalis pes-caprae,* can benefit the digestive system: reducing indigestion, stimulating the appetite, and stopping vomiting.[6] In addition, Oxalis can relieve urinary tract infections,[7] perhaps because of diuretic and astringent qualities.[8] Due to cooling effects, Oxalis leaf decoction may be useful for high fevers,[9] both by quenching thirst and alleviating the fever.[10] Wood Sorrels possess vitamin C, which prevents scurvy, a terrible disease caused by vitamin C deficiency, and benefits the immune system.[11] Wood Sorrels can treat hemorrhages and cleanse the blood.[12]

EXTERNAL USAGE: When applied topically, Wood Sorrels can staunch bleeding due to astringent properties.[13] Oxalis has been known to reduce wounds, swelling, inflammation,[14] skin infections, scrapes, and rashes.[15] These herbaceous plants can reduce mouth ulcers and sores when taken as a gargle.[16]

PREPARATION: Oxalis's internal preparation consists of an infusion, decoction, or juice of the fresh or dried leaves,[17] although use of the entire plant is possible.[18] (See "Sour Grass Lemonade" in "Recipes.") For external application, a cloth or cotton swab saturated with the juice can be manufactured.[19] In addition, juicing this herb and then letting it dehydrate and crystallize will create a Salts of Lemon / Salts of Sorrel substance, which can be applied topically for medicinal purposes.[20]

WARNINGS: Never ingest Salts of Lemon / Salts of Sorrel preparations.[21] Although oxalic acid is totally safe in small quantities, excessive internal usage of Wood Sorrels will have harmful effects on the body. High internal doses may result in digestive or kidney issues,[22] calcium loss in the bones, diarrhea,[23] and less absorption of minerals.[24] Cooking Wood Sorrels will reduce the oxalic acid content in the actual plants, although not necessarily in the resulting infusion.[25] Individuals with rheumatoid arthritis, kidney disease, kidney stones, or gout should avoid any internal use of Sour Grass.[26, 27]

In conclusion, herbal preparations of Sour Grass should be consumed in moderate amounts only.[28]

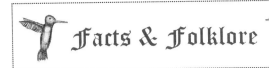

Facts & Folklore

Oxalis pes-caprae is native to South Africa, although this weed has naturalized elsewhere and is difficult to control.[29] Although there is no botanical support for any one true shamrock,[30] this famous symbol of the Irish is believed by some to be an oxalis.[31] Since three was a magical number in the Celtic faith, the shamrock was a sacred plant to the Druids of Ireland, as the shamrock's leaves form a triad.[32] Later, Saint Patrick used the shamrock to establish the Holy Trinity in Ireland.[33]

Wood Sorrels have excellent culinary usage. The aerial parts are refreshing to nibble on trails.[34] Oxalis species are edible raw or cooked, and can be prepared into salads, sauces,[35] soups, and seasonings, contributing a sour flavor to a dish.[36] Wood Sorrel tea makes an excellent "lemon-less lemonade," and was used by some native tribes for that purpose.[37] Boiling the entire Oxalis plant creates an orange dye.[38] Sour Grass flowers make an amazing dye, which is a brighter yellow than even synthetic pigments. Simply gather handfuls of flowers, add a little water, and squeeze out the bright yellow color.

The long, stringy stems of Sour Grass are my favorite cordage material. To prepare the stems, simply pick the abundant stems by the bunch, bruise to release the juices inside, and place on racks for a week away from direct sunlight. The cordage is strong, edible, easy to reverse wrap, and faintly green in color. Sour Grass stems can be gathered with little restraint. Especially after the plant has flowered, collecting the stems does little harm to the plant, since the above ground parts are left to dry out in a couple months anyway.

Where to find it

Sour Grass reveals itself after the first rain in autumn or winter, and continues to thrive until late spring, growing abundantly in Santa Cruz. Sour Grass loves open meadows, trails, hillsides, farmlands, and gardens, and may also grow along the edges of shady, wooded locations. In addition to enjoying the habitats of the Pogonip, Waddell Creek, UCSC meadows, and Wilder Ranch, Sour Grass covers the hillsides by Highway 1 North, teaming up with Wild Mustard (*Sinapis arvensis*) to create giant patches of magnificent, yellow splendor.

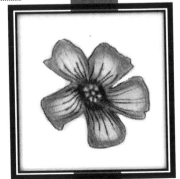

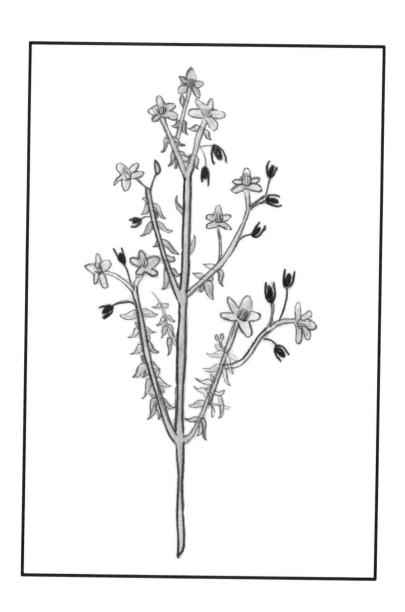

ST. JOHN'S WORT

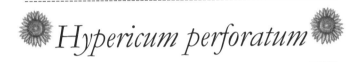

Hypericum perforatum

St. John's Wort is a dainty, one to three foot high plant with bright yellow, five petaled flowers with long stamens. These faintly-scented flowers cluster at the end of oppositely branched stems. The stems are densely covered with small, pointed leaves that contain tiny, translucent spots. The petals, when rubbed between the fingers, produce a red pigment. Hypericum perforatum's *bright yellow flowers bloom only around the summer solstice.*

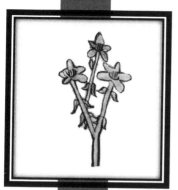

ST. JOHN'S WORT: CURING BURNS AND DEPRESSION

EXTERNAL USAGE: *Hypericum perforatum* is famous for its ability to cure first degree or moderate degree burns.[1] Sores, cuts,[2] and skin ulcers[3] may also be healed by St. John's Wort. Nerve or muscle pain from inflamed joints or tissues can be relieved by *H. perforatum*.[4] St. John's Wort has also been known to help capillary regeneration and yield substantial anti-bacterial effects.[5]

INTERNAL USAGE: Anxiety and depression can be cured with St. John's Wort.[6] People experiencing a loss of confidence, anxious habits, frustration, a feeling of failure, or an overwhelmed mind can feel that their life is restored when consuming the flower tincture.[7] Strong clinical studies have proven St. John's Wort's effectiveness for mild and moderate depression.[8] Mainstream doctors have been known to prescribe this herb.

PREPARATION: Fresh St. John's Wort flowers should be prepared into an oil or salve for external skin rejuvenation.[9] St. John's Wort conveniently infuses in oil when sitting on a sunny windowsill; the double boiler method also works, but is unnecessary. For anxiety or depression, fresh St. John's Wort flowers should be tinctured. Plan on processing the flowers immediately after harvesting, since they wilt quickly and lose their potency.

WARNINGS: Albino cattle that have consumed Hypericum erupt in skin lesions.[10] This caused people to worry that the same reaction would occur in humans. However, external sensitivity to this herb is very rare in humans.[11]

For long-term use of St. John's Wort to alleviate depression, there may be mild side effects.[12] Since this herb is so popular, most health care professionals can offer advice regarding long-term dosage, side effects, and possible interactions with other drugs.

Facts & Folklore

St. John's Wort is a bright and fiery herb, named after St. John, who symbolizes light in Christian customs. The blood-red dots that form on the leaves and stem were believed to mark the day of St. John's beheading.[13] St. John's Wort has been used in divination, and this herb was believed to banish evil spirits and influences, providing luck and protection.[14] St. John's Wort is native to Western Asia and Northern Africa, but grows throughout the world. St. John's Wort especially thrived in California and Oregon, and was considered an invasive weed in the mid 1900's, when it covered about 2.34 million acres. In order to reduce this plant's numbers, a specific Australian beetle, found to acquire an appetite for Hypericum species, was brought over intentionally and, by 1957, reduced St. John's Wort's population by 99%.[15]

Where to find it

I was excited to discover Hypericum near Ano Nuevo, and gathered flowers from the massive tangle of the six foot high bushes. However, the flowers did not contain the typical red pigment when the fresh petals were squeezed, and did not turn the oil red when infused. After research, I learned that there are more than 400 species in the Hypericum family, and although this plant was a Hypericum species, it was not St. John's Wort (*H. perforatum*), the only studied and potent variety. The lesson I learned was that it is always important to identify the exact species of a plant before gathering, because it may matter.

Immediately following that experience, I was blessed to see a three-foot high *Hypericum perforatum* plant growing on a slope into a dried riverbed at Henry Cowell. This was proof enough that this potent herb grows in Santa Cruz County. This herb is currently an invasive weed in the Sierra Nevada foothills, and has historically adapted well to Santa Cruz County. While hiking in June, keep a lookout for St. John's Wort's cheery yellow flowers!

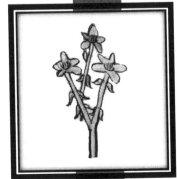

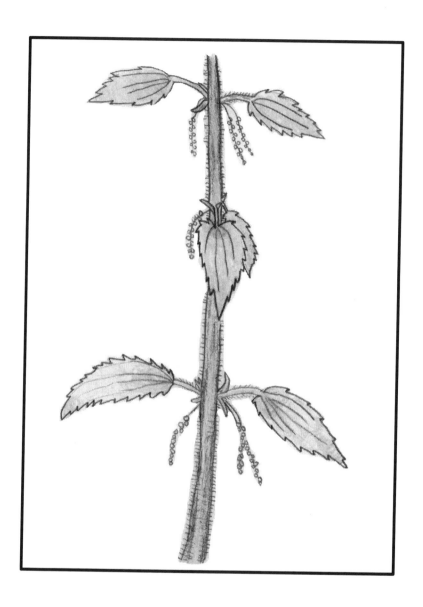

STINGING NETTLE

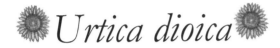

Urtica dioica

Stinging Nettle is a two to six foot high perennial herb with heart shaped, serrated leaves. The stem and leaves are covered with skinny hairs. When the hairs make contact with the skin, a sharp pain is felt, following with minutes to hours of a lingering tingly sensation. Experiencing the sting is a good way to identify Stinging Nettle, but be careful! Hanging from each set of opposite leaves are lightly colored spirals of seeds and flowers.

STINGING NETTLE: DECREASING BLEEDING AND RELIEVING ACHING MUSCLES

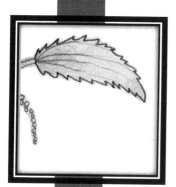

Stinging Nettle appears to be an unwanted, harmful weed, yet that is just a disguise. When protruding outwards, the stinging hairs can penetrate the skin and release histamine, acetylcholine, and serotonin into the body,[1] but once the leaves are mashed, infused, tinctured, dried or powdered, the stinging properties are neutralized and *Urtica dioica* can be safely consumed.

INTERNAL USAGE: Internally, Stinging Nettle can decrease blood flow, due to this herb's astringency. Stinging Nettle can cure bleeding of the digestive system, lungs, or bladder, in addition to uterine bleeding, excessive bleeding around menopause, and post-partum blood.[2] Internal bleeding may signify a deeper problem, in which case one should be looked at by a doctor, but if the bleeding is not serious, Stinging Nettle can be employed.[3] Stinging Nettle is a menstrual-safe diuretic and astringent,[4] enhancing renal function and stopping urinary tract infections, kidney or bladder stones, and prostate inflammation.[5]

EXTERNAL USAGE: The act of whipping oneself with Stinging Nettle, called "urtification" after the scientific name, is surprisingly beneficial to the body. Stinging Nettle's sting can cure arthritis and aching muscles, give feeling to a numb area, and decrease the original pain.[6] *Urtica dioica* can also treat joint pain, sprains, and insect bites.[7] Stinging Nettle seeds can be prepared into a vinegar or oil and applied directly to the hair, in order to increase hair growth and add gleam to the hair and skin.[8, 9]

Stinging Nettle is nutritious, and can be dried and prepared into a powdered superfood,[10] or eaten fresh as a delicious pesto. Stinging Nettle is high in chlorophyll, magnesium, Vitamin C, iron, and protein.[11]

PREPARATION: Stinging Nettle's fresh or dried leaves, in addition to the roots and seeds, should be prepared into an infusion or tincture. The fresh leaf infusion, the most effective internal preparation, is vitamin and mineral rich and delicious.[12] (See "Stinging Nettle Lemonade" in "Recipes," my all-time favorite beverage.) For external preparation, try urtification. I am sure that your sibling or child would be delighted to whip you with a Stinging Nettle stock!

WARNINGS: Never apply Stinging Nettle to an open wound.[13]

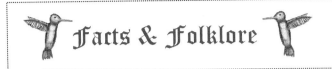

Facts & Folklore

Stinging Nettle stems have long, stringy fibers that I enjoy preparing into strong, green cordage. In addition to cordage, Stinging Nettle fibers have been used for nets, shelters, and a strong substitute for cotton, dating back to 3000 BC.[14] Stinging Nettle has been eaten for its superb nutritional advantages, and was prepared into a green dye for cloth. Stinging Nettle's internal medicinal uses and urtification have been common for thousands of years.[15]

 # Where to find it

Stinging Nettle thrives in shady or partially shady ecosystems such as dried riverbeds, riverbanks, and forests. Places I have gathered Stinging Nettles include Henry Cowell, Grey Whale Creek, and Rancho Del Oso, where this plant grows especially abundantly. This tough perennial herb also grows along the San Lorenzo River, Old San Jose Road region, the Market Street Canal, Point Lobos, Fall Creek, and the Pogonip.

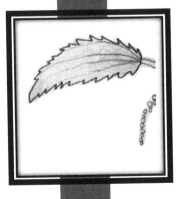

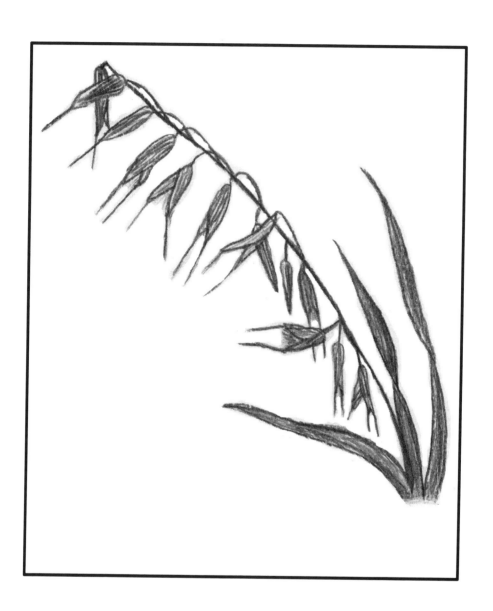

WILD OATS

 Avena fatua, Avena sativa

Wild Oats are two to four foot high grasses that wave in the breezy meadows, with husked seeds hanging off the upper portion of the tall, skinny stems. In winter, Avena fatua sprouts its skinny, pointed leaves, resembling many other grasses. In spring, this herb produces clusters of green oats that contain a white, milky substance. Towards the middle of summer and into autumn, this grass turns crispy and brown as it dries, creating the golden color associated with meadows.

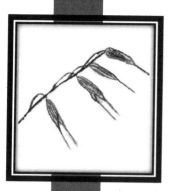

WILD OATS: SOOTHING THE NERVOUS SYSTEM

Avena fatua and *Avena sativa*, the common oat, are both medicinal in the same ways. *Avena barbata*, another species that exists in California, is not legitimate for medicine.[1]

INTERNAL USAGE: Wild Oats are equipped with sedative properties, which can help with mild insomnia,[2] anxiety,[3] depression,[4] emotional or physical exhaustion, and the withdrawal of certain drugs.[5] Since Wild Oats are known to soothe the nervous system and brain, this herb has been known to increase sexual function and desire.[6] Wild Oats might replenish the bones, hair, nails, and skin, due to high contents of silica.[7]

EXTERNAL USAGE: Externally, a bath or soak with Wild Oats can be useful for eczema and irritated,[8] dry, or inflamed skin.[9]

PREPARATION: Gather the seeds in the spring, when they possess the white, milky substance.[10] Gripping the stem below the oats and dragging your hand in an upwards motion releases all the seeds into your hand at once. Fresh Wild Oat seeds can be prepared into a tincture or infusion, while infusions of the dried seeds, stems, and leaves are also practiced.[11]

WARNINGS: Oats may irritate acne, while some *Avena* species can result in asthma or hay fever.[12] Although Wild Oats do not contain gluten, some individuals might be sensitive to the avenins in oats.[13]

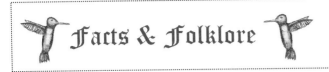

Facts & Folklore

The majority of the non-native plants now naturalized throughout California, including Wild Oats, were initially from the Mediterranean and North African regions.[14] Livestock such as cattle, sheep, and horses were first introduced to California's prairies by the Spanish in 1769.[15] Non-native plants, which were spread both intentionally and accidentally, thrived as soon as these animals overgrazed the native perennial grasses.[16] Wild Oats and other exotic plants introduced during the mission period (1769-1824) drastically and quickly transformed California's original grasslands, creating what was known as "the most spectacular biological invasion worldwide."[17] *Avena fatua* was found in adobe bricks in the oldest parts of the missions' walls.[18] *Avena fatua* seeds are edible and nutritious. After *Avena fatua* was first introduced to California's grasslands, the Cahuillas,[19] a Native American tribe that lived in Southern California,[20] parched the oats and ground them into flour and mush, a practice continued to this day.[21] *Avena sativa* is the cultivated oat prepared into rolled oats and oatmeal, and also as livestock feed.[22] Oats are very nutritious, containing calcium, magnesium, chromium, silica, and more.[23]

Where to find it

Wild Oats comprise the very definition of the word "meadow." *Avena fatua* is the main component of every Santa Cruz meadow and field, growing abundantly. Wild Oats grow in the UCSC meadows, the Pogonip, Arana Gulch, Schwan Lake, Wilder Ranch, Grey Whale Ranch, behind the Santa Cruz Gardens neighborhood, the meadows behind Blue Ball Park, as well as wild gardens and suburban regions. Since this herb is so ubiquitous, one will inevitably come across Wild Oats.

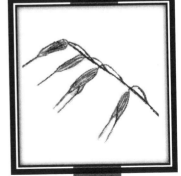

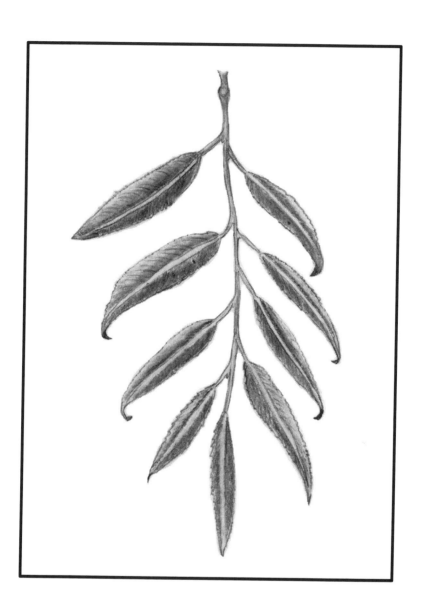

WILLOW

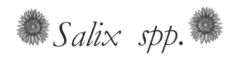

Salix spp.

Willow is a ten to twenty foot high tree with brownish-green bark and leathery, pointed, green leaves with light undersides. In spring, flexible, bendy, green saplings sprout leaves that stick out in every direction. In summer, the leaves turn a darker green, often assembling in a flatter arrangement. Willow, along with its relative Cottonwood, produces rooting hormones on each branch, so if a branch sticks in the ground face up or down, it will become a new tree over time. This is an ingenious adaptation, as a branch floating downstream will naturally take root, thus spreading this tree's range.[1] In the spring and early summer, Salix reproduces by fuzzy, white catkins that carry fluffy seeds. The Willow seeds blow away in the breeze, until they find a spot to propagate.

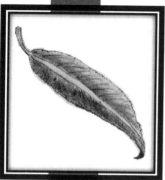

WILLOW: REDUCING PAIN AND FEVER

INTERNAL USAGE: People have known the uses of Willow, and extracted powerful medicine from the bark, since the time of Hippocrates in 400 BC, when people chewed on Willow bark to cure inflammation and fever.[2] Willow has been used since that time as an internal anti-inflammatory, pain reliever, and treatment for headaches, back pain, osteoarthritis, toothaches, and infected gums.[3] The constituent salicin was extracted from Willow bark to create the first aspirin.[4] In addition to salicin, which reduces fevers and pain, other components give this herb anti-oxidant, immune boosting, and anti-microbial qualities.[5] Although there may be multiple *Salix* species in Santa Cruz, all Willows have identical medicinal properties.[6,7] However, not all species accumulate a substantial quantity of salicin.[8] Although Willow is useful towards reducing fever, inflammation, and pain, unlike aspirin, Willow is not helpful as a blood thinner.[9]

EXTERNAL USAGE: The astringent tannins in *Salix* can create an acne treatment.

PREPARATION: To prepare this herbaceous tree, use the fresh or dried chopped stem and bark in a decoction or tincture, or simply chew on the bark directly.[10]

WARNINGS: It is suggested that you should not take *Salix* if you have kidney or liver issues, asthma, diabetes, gout, hemophilia, gastritis, or stomach ulcers and stomach sensitivities. Do not take Willow bark if you are pregnant or allergic to salicin.[11]

𝔉acts & 𝔉olklore

The myths surrounding Willow originated from the characteristics of this tree. Because of this herb's growth in damp places and riverbanks, Willow is associated in ancient Greek mythology with water-magic and the moon, and is featured in myths with Hecate and Helice.[12] Orpheus the poet brings Willow boughs, along with his lyre that was made of Willow wood, down to the underworld.[13] The drooping branches of Willow species such as the weeping willow have been known to symbolize grief, mourning, and sorrow.[14] Because Willow grows quickly, and branches can root into new trees, Willow symbolizes growth and immortality in Chinese culture. [15] Willow was one of the most significant trees to many Native American tribes. The diversity of uses across North America is extraordinary.[16] Because Willow saplings are straight but flexible, I have used them for many projects, including basketry and arrows.

 # Where to find it

Willow trees sprout anywhere possible. I have observed Willow trees at the Arboretum, Arana Gulch, the Santa Cruz Yacht Harbor, Waddell Creek, along most of the San Lorenzo River, and on roadsides. Willow grows in open areas, often in damp soil near a water source, but not necessarily. Willow also creates a unique coastal habitat of its own. In most locations in Santa Cruz County, Willow is the intermediary ecosystem between the beach and inland habitats of meadow or forest.

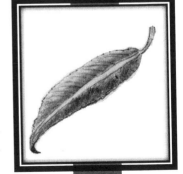

Individual species of Willow are difficult to identify because there are variations within species and they often hybridize.[17] Uses remain the same.

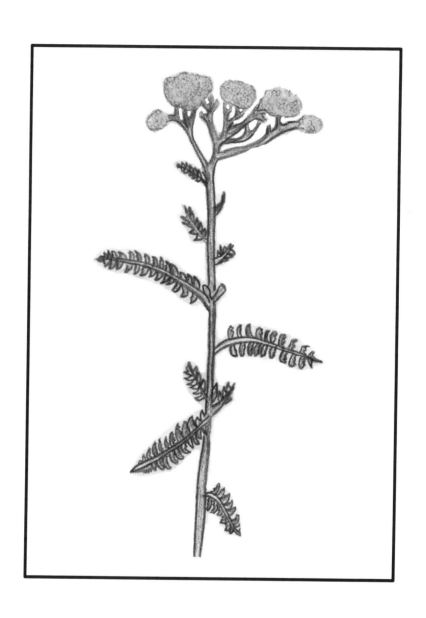

YARROW

 Achillea millefolium

Yarrow is a one to one and a half foot high perennial herb with lacy and feathery leaves that cluster at the base of the plant and travel up the stems. At many times of the year, all that exists of Yarrow is a cluster of lacy leaves. In spring and summer, Achillea millefolium *produces flat, carpet-like tufts of white flowers that seem to hover above the skinny, stiff stems. Yarrow flowers can occur in colors other than white, but those ornamental varieties are not as potent as the wild, white flowered type.[1] Yarrow leaves and flowers smell and taste spicy, but have a bitter aftertaste.*

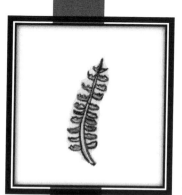

YARROW: STAUNCHING BLEEDING WOUNDS

EXTERNAL USAGE: *Achillea millefolium* is an exceptional wound healer, releasing anti-microbial, astringent,[2] anti-inflammatory,[3] and analgesic properties.[4] Yarrow is most commonly known for its wondrous power in staunching bleeding wounds, due to hemostatic and astringent actions.[5] Yarrow can decrease the swelling in inflamed cuts and wounds,[6] and be beneficial towards burns, bruises, eczema, and ulcers, in addition to reducing blood flow.[7]

INTERNAL USAGE: Internally, Yarrow's astringent and hemostatic properties can stop internal bleeding[8] such as nosebleeds, bleeding stomach ulcers,[9] hemorrhage from wounds, bleeding in the respiratory and urinary systems, as well as bowel and uterine blood.[10] In addition, Yarrow is a circulatory stimulant and also may reduce vein inflammation and thrombosis and lower blood pressure.[11] Yarrow's bitter characteristics aid in digestion and stimulate the appetite, while the astringent tannins may help with intestinal hemorrhage, diarrhea and dysentery.[12] In addition, *Achillea millefolium* is an anti-spasmodic, benefiting the digestive system by relieving cramps, gas, colic, and dyspepsia.[13] Because of diuretic,[14] astringent, anti-bacterial,[15] and anti-inflammatory qualities, Yarrow can relieve urinary complaints such as bladder infections, cystitis,[16] stones, and irritable bladder.[17] Yarrow can also stimulate the kidneys as a diuretic.[18] Internally, Yarrow may work wonders as a diaphoretic,[19] lowering the body temperature and breaking a fever by increasing perspiration.[20] Yarrow potentially assists with colds, sore throats, flu, and coughs when consumed hot.[21]

PREPARATION: In order to extract *Achillea millefolium's* internal qualities, an infusion of the fresh or dried flowers is ideal. A tincture of the whole plant is also practiced,[22] and can be added to hot water or taken directly. For external usage, create a leaf or flower poultice and apply directly, or saturate the inflicted skin with tinctures or infusions.[23] However, my favorite external preparation is Yarrow salve, which is a necessary addition to any first aid kit and is especially useful in combination with Calendula and Plantain. (See "All Purpose Salve" in "Recipes.")

WARNINGS: Since Yarrow will rapidly close a wound, make sure the affliction is entirely clean, so as not to trap material and infection under the skin.[24] Internal use during pregnancy is not recommended.[25]

Facts & Folklore

Achillea millefolium is associated with Achilles, a hero in Greek mythology. Held by his heel, newly born Achilles was submerged by his mother into a bath of Yarrow tea, making him invincible throughout his many battles.[26] It is suggested in the *Iliad* that Achilles treated the bloody knife and sword wounds of his soldiers with Yarrow in the Trojan War, recognized as the first to incorporate this herb's wound-healing properties.[27] In World War I, Yarrow was used when other medicine was scarce in the healing of wounded soldiers.[28] The species *millefolium* means "thousand leaves," referring to the fractal leaflets on each intricate leaf stem.[29] Known to yield spiritual power by the Chinese, dried Yarrow stalks are used in a Chinese process called *i ching*, which serves the purpose of an oracle and answers deep questions,[30] as well as connecting an individual with the harmonious order of the universe.[31]

Where to find it

Yarrow exists in open areas such as fields, meadows, roadsides, chaparral areas, and coastal cliff locations. Yarrow grows in the chaparral habitat of Henry Cowell, the Pogonip, Wilder Ranch, Point Lobos, north coast regions, Rio Del Mar, and along the side of Highway 1.

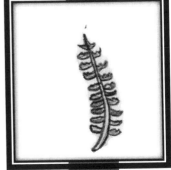

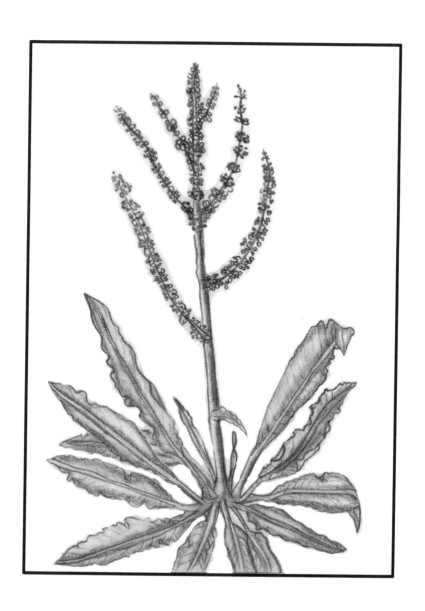

YELLOW DOCK

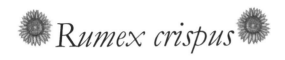

Rumex crispus

Yellow Dock is a two to four foot high perennial weed with large, pointed leaves that jet from the base. Yellow Dock leaves have thick, juicy, green or purple midribs. The edges of each leaf are curled and wavy, or what botanists call "crisped," giving Rumex crispus *its name. Due to these curvy leaves, Yellow Dock is also commonly known as Curly Dock. The leaves of Yellow Dock are edible and delicious, whether raw or cooked in any way that you would prepare spinach. The leaves contain oxalic acid, giving them a sour but palatable flavor. At the beginning of winter, when the leaves are new and fresh, they are tasty and juicy, but they possess an increasingly bitter flavor as spring and summer arrive.[1] Rising way above the cluster of leaves, Yellow Dock extends a tall stalk every spring. Clustered around this stalk are many tiny, green, petal-less flowers with three wings that develop into reddish-brown seeds. The seeds are edible and have been made into flour and other preparations, yet the shell is tough to remove yet distasteful if left.[2] Beneath the soil lies a brown root, which is bright yellow inside, for which the title "Yellow Dock" is derived.*

YELLOW DOCK: ELIMINATING AND DETOXIFYING

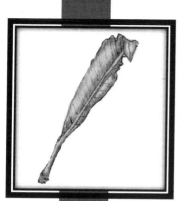

IINTERNAL USAGE: *Rumex crispus* can rid the body of wastes and detoxify. Being a laxative, Yellow Dock can remove waste from the intestines, and due to diuretic qualities, Yellow Dock can eliminate toxins from the bladder.[3] The removal of these wastes prevents buildup in the liver, gallbladder, and blood, improving the body's overall health.[4] Furthermore, Yellow Dock detoxifies by stimulating bile production, assisting with digestion, specifically of fats.[5] Yellow Dock has astringent, antioxidant, and antimicrobial properties.[6] Yellow Dock may help with some blood diseases,[7] anemia, and bleeding in the lungs.[8] Additionally, Yellow Dock is a bitter digestive tonic and can heal sore throats and rheumatism.[9]

EXTERNAL USAGE: Externally, Yellow Dock root can be used as for wounds, sores, rashes, ulcers, skin infections, athlete's foot,[10] hemorrhoids,[11] chronic skin diseases,[12] toothaches, and mouth inflammation.[13]

PREPARATION: The fresh or dried Yellow Dock root can be made into a decoction, syrup, or tincture. All parts of this plant can be used, yet the roots are the most medicinal.[14] Externally, apply a poultice, salve, or powder.[15]

WARNINGS: Overconsumption of Yellow Dock may cause kidney stones to form, since Yellow Dock contains calcium oxalate and oxalic acid. (See "Sour Grass" for more information.) People prone to kidney stones should not consume Yellow Dock, and no one should consume Yellow Dock in excessive amounts due to the risk of kidney stones.[16]

Facts & Folklore

In the Great Depression, when people had no money for food, this plant was sought after and made into salads. Yellow Dock is very nutritious, containing iron, phosphorus, calcium, and loads of vitamin A, C, and protein.[17] Yellow Dock is native to Europe, but naturalized worldwide, where it is considered an invasive weed in around forty different countries.[18] Native Americans made a flour and mush from the seeds, yet only in times of need.[19] A yellow, green, or brown dye can be obtained from the roots.[20]

 # Where to find it

Yellow Dock grows in meadows, fields, roadsides, waste areas, wild gardens, and farmland habitats, in full sun or partial shade. I have seen Yellow Dock thriving at Arana Gulch, Rancho Del Oso, Wilder Ranch, Henry Cowell, the Arboretum, Gray Whale, the Pogonip, Lighthouse Field, the lower San Lorenzo River, and Harkins Slough in Watsonville.

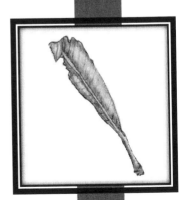

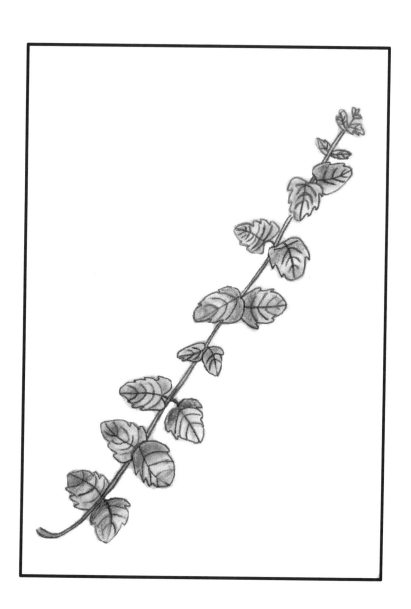

YERBA BUENA

 Clinopodium douglasii

Extending from one to two feet long, Yerba Buena's stem doesn't grow upwards, but trails along the ground. Like all other members of the mint family, Yerba Buena has a square stem and opposite leaves. The thick leaves have serrated edges, and sometimes acquire a tinge of purple on the underside. The leaves are edible and taste spicy like peppermint. However, I prefer to eat the young leaves, since the older and darker ones are tough and not very palatable. Tiny, white, cone-shaped flowers grow close to the stem. Yerba Buena plants grow close together in large patches.

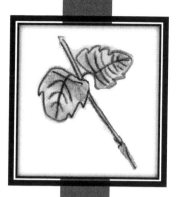

YERBA BUENA: SOOTHING THE DIGESTIVE SYSTEM

INTERNAL USAGE: Yerba Buena means "good herb" in Spanish for a reason. Yerba Buena is a key to digestive health, since this plant is a carminative, and can relieve an upset stomach and soothe digestive membranes.[1] Yerba Buena's anti-spasmodic nature can relieve cramps, diarrhea, constipation, and gas.[2]

In addition, Yerba Buena may treat the kidneys, heal joint pains[3] and sore muscles,[4] and yield diaphoretic properties, relieving fevers.[5]

EXTERNAL USAGE: Externally, Yerba Buena may lessen insect bites.[6] When held in the mouth, a poultice can relieve toothaches.[7]

PREPARATION: Although one can tincture this herb, I strongly recommend infusions with fresh or dried Yerba Buena leaves because of the delicious flavor and fragrance. Munching directly on Yerba Buena leaves can also provide digestive relief. A fresh or dried compress or fresh poultice can be used for external application. [8]

WARNINGS: No cautions known.

𝔉acts & 𝔉olklore

Before San Francisco was founded, a settlement formed at that location called Yerba Buena, named after this scented plant.[9] Because of city development, the herb Yerba Buena no longer grows in San Francisco, although it thrives all along the west coast, even up to Alaska.[10] Native American tribes used Yerba Buena for medicinal purposes for hundreds of years.[11]

 # Where to find it

Yerba Buena lives in shady or partially shady ecosystems such as forests, growing densely in large patches. Yerba Buena dwells at the Arboretum, Grey Whale Ranch, UCSC meadows, Little Basin, and the Pogonip.

Synonyms for *Clinopodium douglasii* are *Micromeria douglasii* and *Satureja douglasii*.[12, 13] However, the common name Yerba Buena can refer to many plants besides this species, so be sure to identify properly.

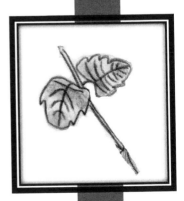

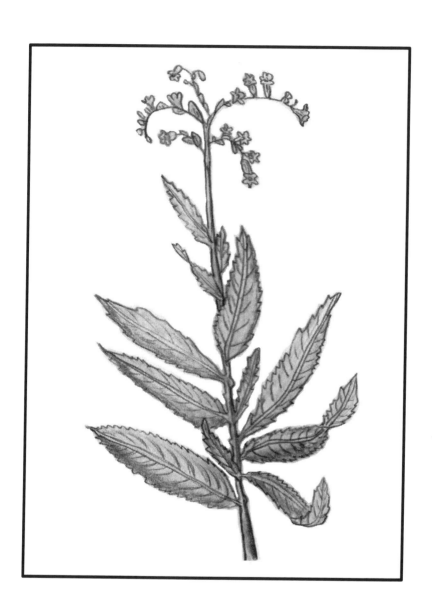

YERBA SANTA

 Eriodictyon californicum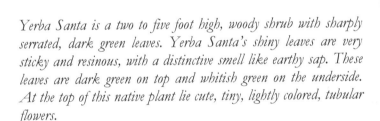

Yerba Santa is a two to five foot high, woody shrub with sharply serrated, dark green leaves. Yerba Santa's shiny leaves are very sticky and resinous, with a distinctive smell like earthy sap. These leaves are dark green on top and whitish green on the underside. At the top of this native plant lie cute, tiny, lightly colored, tubular flowers.

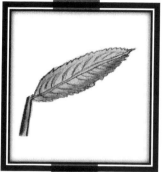

YERBA SANTA: DECONGESTING THE LUNGS AND SINUSES

INTERNAL USAGE: *Eriodictyon californicum* can yield anti-inflammatory, expectorant, anti-spasmodic, anti-microbial, and diuretic properties.[1] As a decongestant and anti-inflammatory, Yerba Santa can assist with lung and sinus conditions with excess mucus and inflammation.[2] Yerba Santa can cure bronchitis, sinus allergies, early stages of moist asthma, a runny nose,[3] irritating dry coughs, whooping cough, and colds.[4] In addition, *Eriodictyon californicum* can be useful towards chronic urethral irritation, gastritis,[5] and chronic rheumatism as a blood purifier.[6]

EXTERNAL USAGE: Yerba Santa can relieve wounds, bruises, sprains, insect bites, and rheumatic pains.[7]

PREPARATION: An infusion or tincture should be prepared from the dried leaves.[8] (See "Yerba Santa Infusion" in "Recipes.") A poultice should be prepared for external purposes.[9]

WARNINGS: If consumed in high quantities, Yerba Santa can cause one's membranes to dry up excessively.[10]

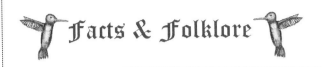
Facts & Folklore

The name Yerba Santa means "Saintly Herb" in Spanish. However, there are a number of herbs that are completely different species, all under the name "Yerba Santa."[11] To avoid confusion, recognize this plant as *Eriodictyon californicum* and learn to identify this plant accurately.[12] In the Mexican magical arts, called *curandismo*, it is believed that Yerba Santa, along with other sacred herbs in a bouquet, will bring spiritual protection to the home.[13] This magical herb has a history of use as an altar offering.[14] Native Americans in the western United States conducted herbal practices of this plant in similar ways as those today.

Where to find it

Yerba Santa thrives in chaparral habitats in Santa Cruz and also does well on mountain ridges and slopes. The main place that I have seen this plant is at the Bonny Doon Ecological Reserve, where it covers the chaparral ecosystem. Yerba Santa also grows in the chaparral areas of Nisene Marks, Henry Cowell, and Little Basin. Since the leaves are often covered in black fungus, pick carefully when harvesting this herb.

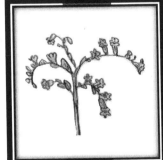

RECIPES

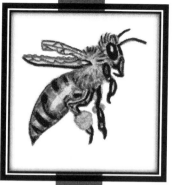

INTRODUCTION TO HERBAL PREPARATION

Wildcrafting medicinal plants from the local landscape and preparing them into your very own herbal medicines is one of the most rewarding and inspiring ways to appreciate the natural world.

It is important to clarify that pharmaceutical drugs are without question the best choice for life-threatening problems. However, for less serious complaints such as coughs, digestive issues, and external wounds, homemade herbal recipes can treat these acute problems effectively. Even if you do not think preparing herbal medicines are your savvy, I heartily encourage experimentation—you may change your mind! Not only do homemade herbal recipes give an unexplainable satisfaction, but they cost almost nothing to produce, in contrast to the extremely expensive medicines at health food stores, especially in the syrup and tincture markets.

Although every herbal recipe has its own precise steps, there are a few standard elements to keep in mind when making any medicinal preparation:

Drying: Although many recipes work best with fresh plants, since they are usually more potent, many herbs can be dried for storage and later preparation. Therefore, knowing how to dry and preserve plants is a very useful skill.

There are several methods to dry herbs. All of these methods should be done outside of direct sunlight, since sunlight can deplete the constituents. One way to dry small plant parts is to simply place them in an open paper bag for a few days. In addition, one can manufacture a flat drying rack out of a cardboard box and allow the plants to dry for as long as needed. Lastly, one can bundle herbs in a bouquet using a rubber band or twine, and hang upside down until dry. The size and height of the plants used will naturally determine which method is most convenient. In addition to these traditional methods, one can purchase a dehydrator, an appliance specifically designed to suck the moisture out of plants.

Straining: Most herbal preparations need to be strained after the components are fully extracted. Straining thoroughly is essential to prevent fermentation, particularly in syrups and oils. To do this, cut a square of cheesecloth and put it on the lid of a glass jar, forming a shallow pocket for the herbs to collect. Wrap a rubber band tightly around the lid to hold the cheesecloth firmly in place, and then pour the liquid into the jar below. Most herbal recipes recommend squeezing out every last precious drop, yet truthfully, the effort and mess required for straining that last eighth of a cup may not be worth the trouble. For maximum product, carefully remove the cheesecloth and herb bundle, squeeze out the last drops, and discard. An easier method is to find a stainless steel tea strainer that fits seamlessly onto your jar lids, and is sturdy enough not to slip while you pour.

Labeling: You think you will always remember what that jar of oddly colored liquid resting on your shelf contains, but trust me, you will forget. Label everything immediately after preparation, recording the necessary information on an adhesive label. Documentation should include: all ingredients used (include scientific names to limit confusion); the date prepared; and the location of harvest.

Although this may seem unnecessary, you will be surprised by how easy it is to forget details from even a few weeks ago. For remedies that take several weeks to infuse, label the temporary container and then transfer the message onto the final jars. In addition to labeling the containers, I also recommend keeping a recipe log in a journal—it is satisfying to record the process and have written recipes to show for it.

Storage: Unused tincture bottles, empty salve and chapstick containers, and glass Mason jars can be purchased at the Herb Room on Mission Street and local health food stores. It is best to store your herbal medicine collection in airtight containers in a cool, dark location. This is because light, heat, and air can deteriorate the components and thus compromise the final result. Create an organized storage space somewhere accessible in the house, yet still refrigerate the less stable remedies to increase their longevity.[1]

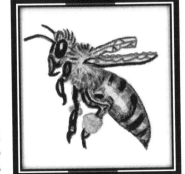

I hope the following recipes empower you to seek natural healing from the earth and you continue to discover the magic that the natural world has to offer!

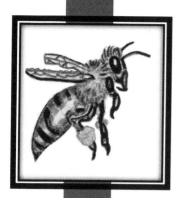

BASIC INTERNAL RECIPES

INFUSIONS

The act of brewing infusions, also known as teas, is an ancient practice that is still popular to this day. An infusion, one of the simplest and most instantly rewarding recipes, is a combination of fresh or dried herbs and boiling hot water. Drinking infusions can be relaxing, comforting, delicious, and healing to the body.[1] Although infusions can treat acute illnesses, they may also prove beneficial when dealing with long term problems, providing a gradual yet continuous treatment.[2]

Leaves and flowers, in addition to some fruits and seeds, are typically used in an infusion, especially when containing volatile oils. To prepare an infusion, begin by boiling water in a pot or tea kettle. Once the water boils, remove from heat. Place the herbs in the pot (either in a tea bag or loose) to infuse. Although the amount differs from herb to herb, a standard infusion has one teaspoon dried herbs or two tablespoons fresh herbs for every cup of water.[3]

Cover and allow the mixture to steep for at least twenty minutes,[4] an important step since steeping allows the constituents to thoroughly infuse into the water. Although the typical cup of tea is nice, for medicinal purposes prepare infusions by the quart.[5] Infusions can be drunk hot, allowed to cool, or consumed chilled on hot days. Although excellent for instant usage, infusions will not stay fresh for longer than a day, even if refrigerated.[6] Since this remedy is short-lasting, a new batch of herbal tea should be brewed and drunk daily when attempting to cure chronic diseases or simply maintain a healthy body.[7]

I heartily recommend experimenting with infusions when first beginning herbal experimentation. I specifically suggest infusing the local herbs: Sour Grass, Stinging Nettle, Yerba Buena, Wild Oats, and Pineapple Weed.

DECOCTIONS

Differing from the infusion method, a decoction demands that the herbs are actually boiled in water, as opposed to simply steeped. Preparing a decoction allows tougher plant parts such as roots, stems, bark, and some fruits and seeds to release chemical components that would otherwise not extract into an infusion. To prepare a decoction, add herbs to water in a pot and bring to a boil. With a tight fitting lid, let the mixture simmer for around twenty minutes, or until infused to your satisfaction. Strain the medicine and drink immediately, or let the un-strained solution sit for a stronger decoction. Keep refrigerated, but know that the decoction will still ferment if kept longer than a day. Tough, fibrous plant parts can be decocted several times before discarding.[8] In order to utilize both types of plants in one water preparation, prepare a decoction, remove from heat, and let the tender plant pieces steep as an infusion.[9]

TINCTURES

A tincture is a concentrated alcohol extract of herbs. Tinctures are some of the handiest and most convenient remedies, since they will last for numerous years and are easy to make, store, and consume.[10] To manufacture a tincture, simply place small, fresh or dried herb pieces in a glass pint or quart jar, cover with alcohol, and screw on the lid. When using fresh herbs, a 1:2 ratio of herbs to alcohol should be used, while dried herbs demand a 1:4 or 1:5 proportion. Let the mixture sit in a cool dark place for four-to-six weeks, the longer the better.[11] It is very important to shake the mixture daily, in order to discharge the constituents from the plants. Once fully infused, strain and pour into tincture bottles with droppers and storage jars. Take one or two droppers' worth of tincture or dilute with water. Be sure to use alcohol with at least 80 – 100 proof (40% - 50%). Although brandy tinctures taste slightly better, I like using vodka as my alcohol, primarily because this clear liquid will acquire beautiful earthy colors as the weeks go by. For external tincture preparations, stronger alcohols such as Everclear can be utilized. Extremely concentrated alcohol like Everclear, 95% (190 proof), are not legally sold in California, but can be acquired in states such as Oregon.

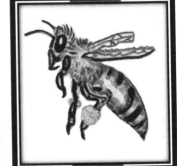

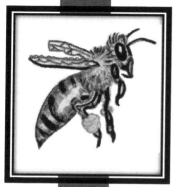

VINEGARS

Medicinal vinegars feature herbs infused in a vinegar solution. For herbal vinegars, the herbs can be added directly into the vinegar or as a decoction and vinegar combination.

For decoction vinegars, create a decoction with herbs. Bring to a boil and, once fully infused, strain out the plants. While still hot, add equal parts Apple Cider Vinegar and pour into the desired bottles. Keep refrigerated. The remedy should last around six months to a year.

The other vinegar recipe combines fresh or dried herbs and the vinegar in a jar. Let the mixture sit for at least a month before straining. Shake daily. The strained vinegar can last six months to a few years if stored in the refrigerator or a cool, dark place.[12] There is a minor caution about vinegars: when using metal jar lids, vinegar will cause the lid to rust. In order to solve this problem, cover the top with a square of wax paper before allowing the infusion process to take place.

A few droppers' worth of infused vinegars can be taken daily. Infused vinegars can also be used in cooking or combined with other ingredients as salad dressings.

SYRUPS AND HONEY INFUSIONS

Fresh or dried roots, bark, fruits, seeds, and other plant parts can generally be made into a syrup or honey infusion. Using honey in herbal recipes not only creates a sweet and delicious potion, but soothes the membranes of the throat and digestive tract, and act as an effective preservative.[13]

Syrups are ideal for high-moisture herbs. To manufacture a syrup, first prepare a strong herbal decoction. Bring herbs and water to a boil and let the mixture simmer until infused to your satisfaction, or at least twenty minutes. Strain the decoction and, while still warm, add equal parts raw bee honey. Shake and stir until combined. Be aware that pouring boiling hot water into glass jars can cause cracking. (Placing a metal utensil in the glass jar can conduct the heat away from the vulnerable glass and might prevent breakage.) Consume by the spoonful a few times per day, or stir into teas, mix into beverages, dilute in water, or dribble atop desserts.[14]

These syrups require constant refrigeration, and sadly enough will last no longer than five months. To further preserve syrups, you can add alcohol: one half cup of 100-proof grain alcohol for every two cups syrup. However, this makes the taste less enjoyable, and I personally prefer to simply acknowledge the fleeting nature of syrups and surrender to making more when necessary.

You may also infuse low-moisture herbs directly in honey for an infused honey preparation. Cut medicinal plants into small pieces and add to the honey (any herbs-to-honey ratio is fine). One way to infuse the honey is to simply let the herbs sit in the honey for around a month. However, in order to reduce the risk of fermentation, put the herbs and honey into a pot and bring to a very low simmer for at least an hour or two. Make sure the mixture does not froth and boil. If the herbs are tasty, leave them in the final honey preparation; otherwise, strain the honey while still warm. Take spoonfuls of this tasty honey when needed, or stir into herbal teas. The advantage of directly infused honey preparations is that they can last for several years and do not need to be refrigerated, since there is no decoction involved.

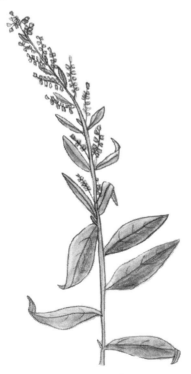

Mugwort in flower

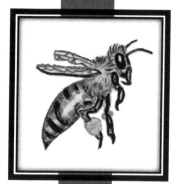

SPECIFIC INTERNAL RECIPES

ARALIA HONEY

Once you have found the desired plant, dig with a stick until you hit the tough, thick Aralia root. Use a knife to cut off two finger-sized chunks from the root system, being especially sure to thank this extraordinary plant. What is nice about harvesting Aralia root is that, if done carefully, you can acquire a substantial amount of root without causing too much permanent damage to the entire plant.

To prepare the roots, remove the dirt and dice into small chunks. One cannot simply brush off the soil; try scrubbing with water and carving off the dirty outer layer. Although fresh roots work well, drying the root can make these steps easier, since the root chunks become brittle.

Once you have prepared the roots, there are two ways of making the syrup. The simplest way is to add raw honey and wait a month or so until it infuses. (Any root-to-honey ratio is fine.) The second method is to put your honey and roots in a pot and bring to a very low simmer for at least an hour or two, making sure it does not froth and boil. I prefer to leave my 'candied' roots in the final herbal honey, since they taste delicious, but you can strain them out if you prefer. Pour the honey into the preferred containers and label. Take spoonfuls of the medicinal honey or stir into herbal teas.

BLUE ELDERBERRY SYRUP

Blue Elderberry Syrup is my favorite internal herbal concoction. I have made many batches of Blue Elderberry

Syrup and all have successfully fought against colds while tasting delicious. Creating this herbal remedy is an amazing experience, with a satisfying resulting product.

It feels great making my own Blue Elderberry Syrup, since this tree is usually teeming with berries that will otherwise spoil on the tree. In addition, Elderberry products are very expensive when purchased at stores, while Elderberry creations can be made at home for almost nothing.

Gather ripe Elderberries in the summer months. Place a cardboard box or bag below a cluster and use clippers to snip. Six large clusters should produce around a cup of syrup. The next step is time-consuming but necessary. Because the stems contain cyanide, meticulously picking each berry from where it is attached on its cluster is required. This can take several hours, but is definitely worth it. I find picking to be easiest and most precise, but using a fork to comb through the berries may also work.

Once the berries are free from all stems, place them in a colander and rinse completely. Then put the Elderberries in a pot and add enough fresh water to encase the berries by several inches. Bring to a boil and mash the berries on the walls of the pot with a spoon as the decoction heats up. This can speed up the infusing process. Let this concoction simmer for an hour or two, stirring at least three or four times per hour. Let the mixture evaporate until slightly less than the original volume, adding additional water throughout the simmer if it begins to thicken. At this point, the liquid should be turning a rich, dark, purple-red color.

Using cheesecloth, strain out the berries while pouring the sour liquid into several quart jars. Remember, boiling hot liquid can break glass jars. While still warm, combine equal parts raw wildflower honey with the tart decoction. Stir well, label, and taste the warm, delicious potion you have created.

The syrup needs to be kept refrigerated. Sadly enough, Blue Elderberry Syrup will only last around three to five months. You can add alcohol (one half cup 100-proof grain alcohol for every two cups syrup) to increase the longevity slightly, but it will make the taste less enjoyable. I think it is best to just be at peace with the syrup spoiling after a few months. For a more practical, long-term recipe, behold the Blue Elderberry tincture.

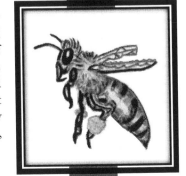

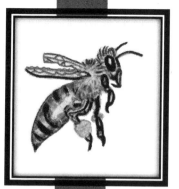

BLUE ELDERBERRY TINCTURE

Although the syrup tastes sweeter and is instantly rewarding, the advantage of creating this red-purple tincture is that it can last for many years and does not need to be refrigerated. After pulling the berries free from their clusters, place them in a jar and mash them up with a spoon. Add vodka in a 1:2 ratio, label, and let the tincture infuse for at least one month. Two to three months is ideal. I have found that the longer the mixture sits before straining, the stronger and darker the resulting tincture will become. Blue Elderberry products are excellent for gifting.

CALIFORNIA POPPY TINCTURE

To prepare a California Poppy Tincture, first uproot numerous California Poppy plants and separate the root from the aerial parts. To prepare the skinny roots, carve off the dirty outer layer with a knife, being careful not to cut into the orange center. Chop the fresh roots into small segments and toss into a pint or quart jar. From the selection of harvested plants, choose some stems, leaves, and flowers, and cut into inch-long pieces. Add these to the jar with the roots and pour brandy or vodka over them with a 1:2 ratio. Let the mixture sit for a month or so and strain.

This remedy should turn a yellow color in vodka. I do not find the taste or smell very pleasant, since this concoction possesses a strongly bitter flavor that lingers on the tongue. However, this can still be an important component in your herbal collection.

HARVESTING AND PREPARING GIANT KELP

Although Giant Kelp gets washed up along most beaches, that kelp is rotting, and is thus not ideal for gathering. Instead, submerge yourself in the ocean where Giant Kelp is visible not too far from the shoreline and snip off several feet from the top portion of the stalk. Make sure to only take what you think will be used. Although snipping off the live stalk may yield a better product, I have wildcrafted detached Giant Kelp drifting in the ocean, which is fine if the kelp is fresh. Cloudy, cool days during low tide are best, since the seaweed is not heating up or drying out. Harvest in the cleanest water possible. Research the water quality of the specific stretch of ocean beforehand; Giant Kelp can contain high levels of cadmium, mercury, lead, or arsenic if those metals are known to occur in that region.

Once the Giant Kelp selection is harvested and transported, rinse the plant in a bucket of water to remove sand. Next, hang the entire plant as you would a clothesline outside in full sunlight and let dry. Giant Kelp will begin to encrust with salt and become stiff as it dries. The drying process might only take a day. It will certainly not take more than a few days to turn the slimy, floppy blades stiff and dry, provided the weather is ideal. Do not over-dry the kelp by keeping it in direct sunlight for an extended period of time. This can cause the kelp to degrade and compromise the quality. In Santa Cruz, I find the weather to be variable, so watch for that "sweet spot" when the kelp should be removed from the sunlight. The medicinal portion of Giant Kelp is the blades attached to the air-filled sacs hanging off the stalk. Once Giant Kelp is completely dry, it is ready to be stored. If properly dried, and placed in an airtight, waterproof container away from any sunlight in temperatures less than 70 degrees Fahrenheit, it should stay nutritionally and medicinally stable ceaselessly.

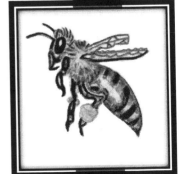

Giant Kelp's dried, salty blades can be further prepared into an infusion, steeped in boiling water for thirty minutes and consumed 3-4 times daily. In addition, Giant Kelp can be taken whole, flaked, powdered, or in capsules.

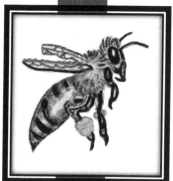

PINEAPPLE WEED INFUSION

Prepare the fresh flower heads using the standard infusion method.

SOUR GRASS "LEMONADE"

Sour Grass infusion tastes very similar to lemonade and is a delicious herbal remedy served hot or chilled.

Pick a handful of Sour Grass leaves and place in a cup or other container. Include the flowers and stems in this recipe if so desired. Add hot water and watch as the plant material immediately drains of its usual color and form, becoming a mush as the mixture infuses. Add raw honey or cane sugar to this infusion, in order to make this beverage truly resemble lemonade.

STINGING NETTLE LEMONADE

Stinging Nettle Lemonade is my favorite beverage. Prepare the leaf infusion using the standard infusion method, which will taste slightly similar to green or black tea. To create a lemonade beverage, add lemon juice and raw honey or cane sugar. Stinging Nettle Lemonade has much more flavor than regular lemonade, which is diluted with plain water. Strain, but enjoy eating the flavorful and nutritious cooked leaves. The stinging qualities of nettles will neutralize when added to hot water, so the leaves are like any flavorful steamed green.

Although a cup of tea is nice, a quart of Stinging Nettle infusion should be used for medicinal purposes.

REDWOOD INFUSION

Collect Redwood needles or cut the end off a Redwood branch adorned with needles. Let the needles dry away from direct sunlight, using a hanging method if the needles are on a branch. The drying process will take at least three weeks. The Redwood needles should be crisp and brittle by the end, yet still possess a pale green color. Surprisingly, the fresh needles do not infuse as well as when dried.

For an infusion, combine the needles with boiling water and steep. I enjoy the evergreen taste and relaxing effect of drinking this elixir.

WILD OATS INFUSION AND TINCTURE

Prepare the fresh oats using the standard infusion and tincture methods. Fresh Wild Oats are more potent than dried ones.

YERBA BUENA INFUSION

Prepare the fresh leaves using the standard infusion method.

YERBA SANTA INFUSION

Yerba Santa Infusion fits the standard infusion preparation; combine leaves with hot water and steep. Although preferred dry, I have infused the fresh leaves with fine results; there is usually not much difference in water content in these waxy leaves.

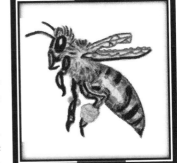

When adding high quantities of leaves to the infusion, the resinous substances will cause the liquid to turn opaque white, resembling milk. The infusion is increasingly bitter and unpalatable the more concentrated, so experiment cautiously.

Lastly, beware that the waxy resin in the leaves can stick to the inside of your cup, which is impossible to clean. Therefore, I advise using a disposable cup for this remedy.

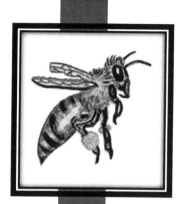

BASIC EXTERNAL RECIPES

HERBAL OILS AND SALVES

There are two ways to manufacture herbal oil. One option is to combine the herbs and oil in a glass jar, and let them solar infuse in a sunny spot for at least two weeks. There is some risk of the oil going rancid and the herbs molding. Some herbs love this cold infusion method, such as St. John's Wort.

On the other hand, some herbs infuse better with the following heat preparation, since they have a sizable moisture content and are more prone to molding, such as Calendula. Heat infusion, my preferred oil recipe, consists of utilizing heat from a stove to infuse herbs in a double boiler method.

Cut the herbs into small pieces and place them in a Pyrex glass container. To use this double boiler method, take the pan filled with herbs and cover with an inch or two of extra virgin olive oil. Rest the pan on the brim of a pot that has a few inches of water inside. Bring to a boil, so the evaporating steam will heat the oil quickly. The temperature of the oil has to maintain a certain balance: it needs to get mildly warm, so that the herbs can infuse in the oil properly, yet the oil cannot overheat and bubble, or else you will fry your herbs. Repeatedly test the temperature with a utensil by dripping the oil onto the back of your hand. Continue heating for one to two hours (the longer the infusion process, the better the result, if kept at a low temperature). Remove from heat and strain the hot, herbal oil into a jar or other temporary container, discarding the diminished herbs. The oil should be unique in smell and appearance at this point, no longer resembling ordinary olive oil.

A salve is an herbal oil combined with beeswax, creating an ointment with a thick consistency that can be applied to the skin directly. A balm is a fragrant ointment, such as a salve with a fragrance added.

Most of us have used lip balm, also called chapstick, without realizing that it is something that can easily be made at home. Not only are salves easier to apply to the skin than oils, but salves have a greater longevity than herbal oils alone. Beeswax is a natural preservative, and salves, if stored correctly, can last for a couple years.

Turning the herbal oil into salve requires melting beeswax into the oil using a double boiler method. If not immediately preparing a salve, store the oil in a cool dark place. Remember to check the herbal oil for rancidity before using. The amount of time it takes to liquefy the beeswax depends on how fine the beeswax pieces are. Grating the beeswax with a cheese grater will cause it to dissolve quickly, while large chunks take longer to disappear. (Designate a cheese grater for this purpose, since beeswax is difficult to completely remove.) Adding the perfect amount of beeswax is a key step in producing a satisfactory result, since both excessively oily and excessively hard salves are inconvenient to apply. Rosemary Gladstar recommends adding one-fourth cup beeswax to every cup of oil,[1] while Michael Moore recommends one ounce beeswax for every five ounces of oil.[2] However, I like to test the consistency as the beeswax dissolves. Start with a small amount of beeswax. Dip a chopstick or skewer in the concoction and allow a drop to harden on a surface. When hot, in liquid form, it is impossible to determine what the consistency will be when at room temperature. Add more beeswax and repeat testing until the desired consistency is achieved. I like to add vitamin E oil to my still-liquid salve for extra skin rejuvenation. Once the beeswax is melted to completion, remove from heat, but do the following steps fast, since the liquid will harden into a salve quickly. Pour into the desired containers; although plastic and metal containers work fine, I prefer glass jars. Before allowing the ointment to harden, you may wish to include several drops per jar of an essential oil such as lavender in order to create a pleasantly scented balm. Experiment using your fresh, rejuvenating medicine on the skin immediately.

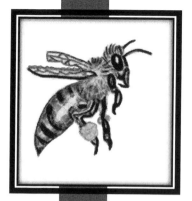

In addition to using salves medicinally, I enjoy applying them as lip balm, so I pour this remedy into empty plastic chapstick containers. A word of caution however: when in direct sunlight, the oils in salves can burn the lips. Adding SPF 15 or higher to chapsticks may solve this problem. Red raspberry seed oil is valued for its sun protection factor, while zinc oxide is another option.[3]

POULTICES

A poultice is an herb paste that can be applied directly on the inflicted area.

To prepare a poultice out of fresh plant parts, such as the leaves, the simplest way is to chew the herbs in your mouth. The plants will release their healing properties as they mix with your saliva. Apply the paste directly on the skin. More hygienic ways to prepare a poultice include pounding, boiling, or steaming the herbs. If using dried herbs, it is necessary to reconstitute them using water or oil.[4]

Generally, to make herbs into a more easily applicable paste and increase the healing actions, mix the herbs with a touch of water, alcohol, oil, Apple Cider Vinegar,[5] green clay (to help draw out infection), or honey (for cuts and rashes).[6]

A poultice should be administered to the skin directly and held for an extended period of time. A poultice is standardly encased in a cotton cloth, but can also be held in place with the hands, although that requires patience. Using a cotton bandage may prove ideal especially since some herbs may irritate the skin when placed directly on a wound.[7]

When starting out manufacturing herbal remedies, I recommend experimenting with poultices. Poultices are the easiest herbal recipe, since they do not require a menstruum (liquid which dissolves the herbs to form a solution) or a fire to heat-infuse the herbs in the menstruum. Poultices are especially convenient on the trail for emergency relief from wounds. In addition to treating many inflictions of the skin, poultices can be held in the mouth to relieve toothaches, mouth ulcers, and sore gums. I have applied poultices of Plantain, Yarrow, Yerba Buena, and Fennel to temporarily reduce the pain of toothaches.

The following herbal recipes are topical liquid preparations. Liquid solutions such as infusions, decoctions, vinegars, and tinctures can have powerful healing effects externally and can be administered as compresses, baths, soaks, gargles, and mouthwashes as described in the subsequent recipes.

COMPRESSES

A compress differs from a poultice in that a compress involves saturating a soft, clean cloth with an infusion or tincture. Place the saturated compress directly on the skin, being sure to keep it continually wet. Cotton balls and cotton swabs make excellent compresses, as well as soft cotton cloth scraps wrapped like bandages. Another acceptable liquid application is simply dripping or misting from a spray bottle and then rubbing into the skin. However, compresses are convenient for long-term application.

For increased medicinal healing, consider wrapping a poultice of solid herbs inside a compress cloth.[8]

BATHS AND SOAKS

Immersing the body in herbal solutions can be a pleasurable and relaxing way of healing the skin. An herbal bath is made by infusing herbs in hot bathwater. You can contain the herbs in a cheesecloth or muslin bag tied around the faucet. Let the herbs steep for a few minutes and then enter your spa, making sure to inhale the fragrant herbal steam deeply and relax.[9] In order to utilize the tougher plant materials, and perhaps create a more concentrated bath, one can prepare a decoction of the roots, bark, etc. by boiling them in water. Let steep, strain, and then add to a full bathtub.[10] In addition, tinctures can be poured into herbal baths. Although a full body medicinal bath is relaxing, there are times when it is not practical, such as when dealing with only one portion of the body. A soak, which is a bath delivered to only that specific body part, can be prepared in any tub. Foot soaks can work well in treating fungal infections such as athlete's foot.[11]

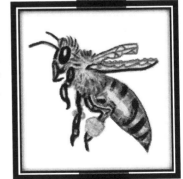

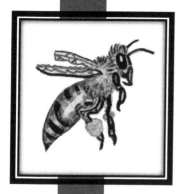

The following herbal preparations can be categorized as external medicines, even though they are to be administered on internal body parts such as the mouth and lungs.

GARGLES AND MOUTHWASHES

Gargles and mouthwashes are infusions, decoctions, or diluted tinctures of astringent herbs swished around and gargled in the mouth. Gargling requires tilting the head back and constantly exhaling through the liquid to prevent swallowing. Deep gargling allows this rinse to reach the upper throat, enabling relief from throat infections. Gargles and mouth rinses can also treat gum inflammation, mouth ulcers, and comfort the mucous membranes of the mouth and throat. Once thoroughly rinsed, one can empty from the mouth or swallow, depending on the herb.[12] I recommend diluted Himalayan Blackberry tincture for gargling, useful for temporarily relieving sore throats.

STEAM INHALATIONS

Steam Inhalations are herbal infusions and decoctions inhaled into the lungs, especially useful for expectorant and antimicrobial herbs.

To prepare a steam inhalation, boil water in a pot. Boiling the herbs in a decoction causes medicinal steam to evaporate from the surface. Once boiling, lean over the pot and breathe through the nose and again through the mouth for several minutes, clearing the nasal passages and soothing the lungs. Placing a towel over the head and shoulders can increase the amount of medicinal steam entering the mouth and nostrils. Inhaling the steam can have a relaxing effect on the body and give off a pleasant aroma.

SPECIFIC EXTERNAL RECIPES

ALL-PURPOSE SALVE: PLANTAIN, YARROW, AND CALENDULA

All-Purpose Salve is my favorite external remedy. Every time I use this salve, I am in awe of how well it works for a vast assortment of topical ailments. The healing properties of Plantain, Yarrow, and Calendula merge together harmoniously to create something miraculous, a salve that seems to heal many acute afflictions of the skin in a short period of time. All-Purpose Salves make excellent gifts. Relatives and friends have been grateful for this salve's skin healing properties.

To create an All-Purpose Salve, harvest many Calendula flowers, clip numerous Yarrow flower heads, and gather Plantain leaves. In addition, I have also added Lavender flowers *(Lavendula officinalis)* to my salve, with great results. Cut the herbs into small pieces in a Pyrex glass container, and fill with extra virgin olive oil. After one or two hours of heating this oil with the double boiler method, this remedy will have a pleasantly bitter smell and dark green color, no longer resembling any normal olive oil. Once you are satisfied with the infusion's progress, remove from heat and strain into a jar. Calendula is prone to molding in the cold-infused method. Therefore, it is important to prepare All-Purpose Salve using the heat infused method.

Turning the herbal oil into salve requires melting beeswax into the oil, again using the double boiler method. After the beeswax is fully dissolved, I like to add vitamin E oil from a few capsules for additional skin rejuvenation. Remove from heat and pour into the desired containers quickly. I like adding an essential oil such as Lavender to this salve to create a pleasantly scented balm. In addition to the medicinal benefits for the skin, I enjoy All-Purpose Salve for chapped lips, and pour this remedy into plastic chapstick containers. However, see caution in "Herbal Oils and Salves."

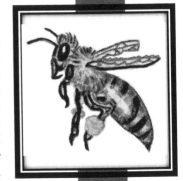

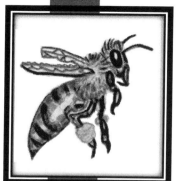

BLUE GUM EUCALYPTUS STEAM INHALATION

Find a Blue Gum Eucalyptus sapling with young leaves, which I prefer, or access a low-hanging branch. Pick a handful or two of these leaves and dry in a paper bag. Once dry, add a small handful of the leaves into a pot of water and bring to a boil. Once boiling, lean over the pot and breathe through the nose and again through the mouth for several minutes to clear the nasal passages and soothe the lungs. The expectorant properties work remarkably; have tissues in arm's reach. Repeat this process at least twice per day when down with a cold, especially shortly before sleep and when congested in the morning.

Blue Gum Eucalyptus is my go-to preparation when I have a head cold, and I find this herb to be an exceptional decongestant. Inhaling the steam has a relaxing effect on the body and gives off a strong yet pleasant smell.

BALM OF GILEAD

Harvest the Cottonwood leaf buds. Be respectful and make sure not to pick too many Cottonwood buds from a single tree. They need them to create new leaves, so spread out your harvest amongst multiple trees. Combine with extra virgin olive oil in a Pyrex glass container. To properly infuse Cottonwood buds, 130 degrees Fahrenheit for 18-24 hours is required. This can be done with some ovens, yet most oven temperatures are not accurate until above 200 degrees Fahrenheit. Cheri Callas, acupuncturist and herbalist, let me borrow her electric pressure cooker called Instant Pot Duo, which had a yogurt making setting at 130 degrees Fahrenheit. This worked beautifully, and was convenient since it did not require my constant attention for 18-24 hours. After straining, I had a powerfully infused oil, which I further combined with beeswax in the double boiler method to produce a magnificent stash of Balm of Gilead.

According to Darren Huckle, an herbalist and acupuncturist, one can also tincture the buds in a high proof alcohol (95%), and combine in a salve when melting the beeswax. A 95% (190 proof) alcohol such as Everclear is not legally sold in California, but can be acquired in states such as Oregon.

HIMALAYAN BLACKBERRY ASTRINGENT

This remedy is great for teenagers with oily skin, and is one that I have found helpful for acne. Himalayan Blackberry is so easy to encounter, and is a medicinal herb often taken for granted and ignored. To prepare this facial astringent, use scissors or clippers to snip the leaves off the vine, enough to stuff a paper bag. You may want to wear gloves, since the vine and leaves are covered in painfully sharp thorns. While the leaves are still fresh, snip each leaflet from its cluster of five. Stack the leaves and cut in small pieces into a jar. The leaves should be stuffed in the jar tightly, but with enough room for vodka to seep into all the cracks and saturate every leaf. Let the vodka tincture infuse for around a month, and then strain out the leaves. To prepare the compress, saturate cotton pads or cotton balls with the tincture. You can saturate many pads at once or before each use. Warning: the black or yellow-brown tincture has a distasteful smell. Therefore, I like to add several drops of Lavender essential oil for a pleasantly-scented cleansing pad. Wipe or lightly dab this compress onto the face once or twice per day. Overuse of astringents can dry out the skin too much, so apply with moderation. Store in a sealed jar to ensure that the cleansing pads do not dry out. One can also pour the tincture into a spray bottle and spritz onto the face. Another way to manufacture this remedy is to create an infusion with the leaves. Let the Himalayan Blackberry leaves steep fully and then combine with your preferred amount of alcohol. If your skin is sensitive to alcohol, you can eliminate it from the recipe and simply use the fresh infusion on the skin. Infusion preparations will not last longer than a day or two, and need refrigeration. Witch Hazel may also prove a good alternative to alcohol remedies.

POISON OAK RINSE: MUGWORT AND HORSETAIL

Harvest the aerial parts from several Horsetail plants and a handful or two of Mugwort leaves. In a pot, cut the fresh Horsetail into small pieces and boil with water as a decoction. Remove from heat and steep the fresh Mugwort leaves. Strain and add equal parts Apple Cider Vinegar. Pour into spray bottles and spritz onto the skin in the event of a Poison Oak rash, or as a preventative if you may have encountered Poison Oak. A tingling sensation may be experienced upon application. Keep refrigerated.

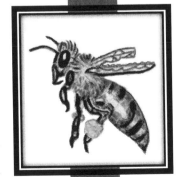

THERAPEUTIC USE LIST

This therapeutic use list in intended as a quick reference guide. Please refer to the individual entries for specific usage information pertaining to your symptoms and possible warnings.

Herbs that tend to be especially effective are in bold.

DIGESTIVE SYSTEM

Fennel
Yerba Buena
Blue-Eyed Grass, Blue Gum Eucalyptus, Calendula, California Bay, California Poppy, Dandelion, Himalayan Blackberry, Horsetail, Mallow, Milk Thistle, Miner's Lettuce, Mugwort, Pineapple Weed, Plantain, Sour Grass, Stinging Nettle, Yarrow, Yellow Dock, Yerba Santa

URINARY SYSTEM

~Bladder infections, kidney stones

Horsetail
Dandelion
Redwood
Blue Gum Eucalyptus, California Tiger Lily, Fennel, Himalayan Blackberry, Mallow, Milk Thistle, Miner's Lettuce, Plantain, Sour Grass, Stinging Nettle, Yarrow, Yellow Dock, Yerba Buena, Yerba Santa

CIRCULATORY SYSTEM

~Cholesterol, blood pressure, anemia, general heart function, hemorrhages

California Tiger Lily
Yarrow
Stinging Nettle
Blue Gum Eucalyptus, Calendula, Dandelion, Himalayan Blackberry, Milk Thistle, Miner's Lettuce, Mugwort, Redwood, Sour Grass, Yellow Dock, Yerba Santa

COLDS AND INFLUENZA

~Coughs, sore throat, general respiratory illnesses, immune boosters

Blue Elderberry
Aralia
Blue Gum Eucalyptus
Calendula, California Poppy, California Tiger Lily, Cottonwood, False Solomon Seal, Fennel, Giant Kelp, Himalayan Blackberry, Horsetail, Mallow, Milk Thistle, Miner's Lettuce, Pineapple Weed, Plantain, Redwood, Stinging Nettle, Willow, Yarrow, Yellow Dock, Yerba Buena, Yerba Santa

FEVERS

Willow
Yarrow
Blue Elderberry, Blue-Eyed Grass, Blue Gum Eucalyptus, Fennel, Mugwort, Pineapple Weed, Sour Grass, Yerba Buena

WOMEN'S HEALTH

~Menstruation, pregnancy, breastfeeding

California Tiger Lily
Stinging Nettle
Blue-Eyed Grass, Calendula, Fennel, Himalayan Blackberry, Mugwort, Pineapple Weed, Yarrow

MENTAL HEALTH

~Depression, insomnia, anxiety, stress, nervine, sedative

St. John's Wort
California Poppy
Wild Oats
Aralia, California Bay, California Tiger Lily, Giant Kelp, Horsetail, Mugwort, Pineapple Weed, Redwood

PAIN RELIEF

~Headaches, joint/muscle pain, arthritis, rheumatism, gout

Willow
California Poppy
Blue Gum Eucalyptus, California Bay, Cottonwood, Dandelion, Himalayan Blackberry, Miner's Lettuce, Mugwort, St. John's Wort

SKIN AFFLICTIONS

~Wounds, rashes, acne, staunching blood flow

Cottonwood
Calendula
Yarrow
Plantain
Blue Gum Eucalyptus, California Bay, Dandelion, False Solomon Seal, Giant Kelp, Himalayan Blackberry, Mallow, Milk Thistle, Mugwort, Pineapple Weed, Redwood, Sour Grass, St. John's Wort, Stinging Nettle, Willow, Wild Oats, Yellow Dock, Yerba Buena, Yerba Santa

ENDNOTES

HERBAL INTRODUCTION

1. "Intermediate Herbal Course." *Herbal Academy of New England,* May 27, 2017. Web. <members.herbalacademyofne.com/course/intermediate-herbal-course>
2. Medicinal Plants." *Wikipedia: The Free Encyclopedia,* May 27, 2017. Web. <https://en.wikipedia.org/wiki/Medicinal_plants>
3. Medicinal Plants." *Wikipedia: The Free Encyclopedia,* May 27, 2017. Web. <https://en.wikipedia.org/wiki/Medicinal_plants>

GUIDE TO HARVESTING FROM THE LANDSCAPE

1. Thayer, Samuel. *Nature's Garden: A Guide to Identifying, Harvesting, and Preparing Edible Wild Plants.* Birchwood, WI: Forager's Harvest Press, 2010. Print.
2. Thayer, Samuel. *Nature's Garden: A Guide to Identifying, Harvesting, and Preparing Edible Wild Plants.* Birchwood, WI: Forager's Harvest Press, 2010. Print.
3. Thayer, Samuel. *Nature's Garden: A Guide to Identifying, Harvesting, and Preparing Edible Wild Plants.* Birchwood, WI: Forager's Harvest Press, 2010. Print.
4. Thayer, Samuel. *Nature's Garden: A Guide to Identifying, Harvesting, and Preparing Edible Wild Plants.* Birchwood, WI: Forager's Harvest Press, 2010. Print.
5. Neddo, Nick. "The Rustic Brayer." *The Organic Artist: Make Your Own Paint, Paper, Pigments, and More from Nature.* Beverly, MA: Quarry Books, 2015. Print.
6. Thayer, Samuel. *Nature's Garden: A Guide to Identifying, Harvesting, and Preparing Edible Wild Plants.* Birchwood, WI: Forager's Harvest Press, 2010. Print.
7. Moore, Michael. *Medicinal Plants of the Pacific West.* Santa Fe, NM: Red Crane Books, 1993. Print.
8. Garms, Gabe. "How to Tell the Difference Between Poison Hemlock and Queen Anne's Lace." Raven's Roots Naturalist School, May 19, 2017. Web. <ravensroots.com/blog/2015/6/26/poison-hemlock-id>
9. Garms, Gabe. "How to Tell the Difference Between Poison Hemlock and Queen Anne's Lace." Raven's Roots Naturalist School, May 19, 2017. Web. <ravensroots.com/blog/2015/6/26/poison-hemlock-id>
10. "How much hemlock would kill you?" The Naked Scientists. May 19, 2017. Web. <thenakedscientists.com/forum/index.php?topic=52195.0>
11. "Poison Oak Rash: Pictures & Remedies." Healthline, May 19, 2017. Web. <healthline.com/health/outdoor-health/poison-oak-pictures-remedies#overview1>
12. "Poison Oak Rash: Pictures & Remedies." Healthline, May 19, 2017. Web. <healthline.com/health/outdoor-health/poison-oak-pictures-remedies#overview1>

GLOSSARY OF HERBAL ACTIONS

1. "Free radicals, antioxidants and functional foods: Impact on human health." *PMC,* May 27, 2017. Web. <ncbi.nlm.nih.gov/pmc/articles/PMC3249911/>

ARALIA

1. Moore, Michael. "California Spikenard." *Medicinal Plants of the Pacific West.* Santa Fe, NM: Red Crane Books, 1993. Print.
2. Moore, Michael. "California Spikenard." *Medicinal Plants of the Pacific West.* Santa Fe, NM: Red Crane Books, 1993. Print.
3. Skenderi, Gazmend. "Spikenard." *Herbal Vade Mecum.* Rutherford, New Jersey: Herbacy Press, 2003. Print.
4. Skenderi, Gazmend. "Spikenard." *Herbal Vade Mecum.* Rutherford, New Jersey: Herbacy Press, 2003. Print.
5. Moore, Michael. "California Spikenard." *Medicinal Plants of the Pacific West.* Santa Fe, NM: Red Crane Books, 1993. Print.
6. Skenderi, Gazmend. "Spikenard." *Herbal Vade Mecum.* Rutherford, New Jersey: Herbacy Press, 2003. Print.
7. Moore, Michael. "California Spikenard." *Medicinal Plants of the Pacific West.* Santa Fe, NM: Red Crane Books, 1993. Print.
8. Moore, Michael. "California Spikenard." *Medicinal Plants of the Pacific West.* Santa Fe, NM: Red Crane Books, 1993. Print.

9. Moore, Michael. "California Spikenard." *Medicinal Plants of the Pacific West*. Santa Fe, NM: Red Crane Books, 1993. Print.
10. Moore, Michael. "California Spikenard." *Medicinal Plants of the Pacific West*. Santa Fe, NM: Red Crane Books, 1993. Print.
11. Skenderi, Gazmend. "Spikenard." *Herbal Vade Mecum*. Rutherford, New Jersey: Herbacy Press, 2003. Print.
12. Moore, Michael. "California Spikenard." *Medicinal Plants of the Pacific West*. Santa Fe, NM: Red Crane Books, 1993. Print.
13. "Spikenard." *Only Foods*, July 29, 2016. Web. <onlyfoods.net/spikenard.html>
14. "Spikenard root." *Mountain Rose Herbs*, July 9, 2015. Web. <mountainroseherbs.com/products/spikenardrootprofile>.
15. "Spikenard." *Wikipedia*, July 29, 2016. Web. <https://en.wikipedia.org/wiki/Spikenard>
16. "Spikenard." *Only Foods*, July 29, 2016. Web. <onlyfoods.net/spikenard.html>
17. Totilo, Rebecca P. "Spiritual Significance of Spikenard." July 9, 2015. Web. <rebeccaatthewell.org/spiritual-significance-of-spikenard>
18. Totilo, Rebecca P. "Spiritual Significance of Spikenard." July 9, 2015. Web. <rebeccaatthewell.org/spiritual-significance-of-spikenard>
19. "Spikenard." *Wikipedia*, July 29, 2016. Web. <https://en.wikipedia.org/wiki/Spikenard>
20. Totilo, Rebecca P. "Spiritual Significance of Spikenard." July 9, 2015. Web. <rebeccaatthewell.org/spiritual-significance-of-spikenard>
21. "Plants Database: Aralia racemosa L. American Spikenard, Legal Status." *USDA Natural Resources Conservation Service*, July 29, 2016. Web. <plants.usda.gov/core/profile?symbol=ARRA>
22. "Species at Risk." *United Plant Savers, Stewards of Healing Herbs*, July 9, 2015. Web. <https://www.unitedplantsavers.org/species-at-risk/5-121-species-risk>

BLUE ELDERBERRY

1. Aniys, Aqiyl. "Elderberry Benefits (*Sambucus Nigra*) – Stop Chest Congestion." *Natural Life Energy*, July 20, 2015. Web. <naturallifeenergy.com/elderberry-benefits-sambucus-nigra-stop-chest-congestion/>
2. "Unit Two: Food Is Medicine." *Herbal Academy of New England Intermediate Herbal Course*, 2015 – 2016. Web. <theherbalacademy.com>
3. Aniys, Aqiyl. "Elderberry Benefits (*Sambucus Nigra*) – Stop Chest Congestion." *Natural Life Energy*, July 20, 2015. Web. <naturallifeenergy.com/elderberry-benefits-sambucus-nigra-stop-chest-congestion/>
4. Aniys, Aqiyl. "Elderberry Benefits (*Sambucus Nigra*) – Stop Chest Congestion." *Natural Life Energy*, July 20, 2015. Web. <naturallifeenergy.com/elderberry-benefits-sambucus-nigra-stop-chest-congestion/>
5. Aniys, Aqiyl. "Elderberry Benefits (*Sambucus Nigra*) – Stop Chest Congestion." *Natural Life Energy*, July 20, 2015. Web. <naturallifeenergy.com/elderberry-benefits-sambucus-nigra-stop-chest-congestion/>
6. Skenderi, Gazmend. "Elder, European." *Herbal Vade Mecum*. Rutherford, New Jersey: Herbacy Press, 2003. Print.
7. Thayer, Samuel. "Elderberry." *Nature's Garden: A Guide to Identifying, Harvesting, and Preparing Edible Wild Plants*. Birchwood, WI: Forager's Harvest Press, 2010. Print.
8. Thayer, Samuel. "Elderberry." *Nature's Garden: A Guide to Identifying, Harvesting, and Preparing Edible Wild Plants*. Birchwood, WI: Forager's Harvest Press, 2010. Print.
9. Thayer, Samuel. "Elderberry." *Nature's Garden: A Guide to Identifying, Harvesting, and Preparing Edible Wild Plants*. Birchwood, WI: Forager's Harvest Press, 2010. Print.
10. Thayer, Samuel. "Elderberry." *Nature's Garden: A Guide to Identifying, Harvesting, and Preparing Edible Wild Plants*. Birchwood, WI: Forager's Harvest Press, 2010. Print.
11. Aniys, Aqiyl. "Elderberry Benefits (*Sambucus Nigra*) – Stop Chest Congestion." *Natural Life Energy*, July 20, 2015. Web. <naturallifeenergy.com/elderberry-benefits-sambucus-nigra-stop-chest-congestion/>
12. Johnson, Rebecca, et al. "Respiratory System." *National Geographic Guide to Medicinal Herbs: The World's Most Effective Healing Plants*. Washington DC: National Geographic Society, 2012. Print.
13. Johnson, Rebecca, et al. "Respiratory System." *National Geographic Guide to Medicinal Herbs: The World's Most Effective Healing Plants*. Washington DC: National Geographic Society, 2012. Print.
14. Thayer, Samuel. "Elderberry." *Nature's Garden: A Guide to Identifying, Harvesting, and Preparing Edible Wild Plants*. Birchwood, WI: Forager's Harvest Press, 2010. Print.
15. Shore, Lynn. "Herbs for Natural Dyeing." *Urban Herbology: Foraging, Growing, and Using Herbs in Amsterdam*, August 4, 2016. Web. <urbanherbology.org/2011/02/06/herbs-for-natural-dying/>
16. Lyons, Kathleen and Mary Beth Cooney-Lazaneo. "Blue Elderberry." *Plants of the Coast Redwood Region*. Boulder Creek, CA: Looking Press, 1988. Print.
17. Lyons, Kathleen and Mary Beth Cooney-Lazaneo. "Blue Elderberry." *Plants of the Coast Redwood Region*. Boulder Creek, CA: Looking Press, 1988. Print.
18. Thayer, Samuel. "Elderberry." *Nature's Garden: A Guide to Identifying, Harvesting, and Preparing Edible Wild Plants*. Birchwood, WI: Forager's Harvest Press, 2010. Print.

BLUE-EYED GRASS

1. Harrison, Marie. "Blue-eyed Grass." *Dave's Garden*, January 6, 2016. Web. <davesgarden.com/guides/articles/view/2492/>

1. Harrison, Marie. "Blue-eyed Grass." *Dave's Garden,* January 6, 2016. Web. <davesgarden.com/guides/articles/view/2492/>
2. Harrison, Marie. "Blue-eyed Grass." *Dave's Garden,* January 6, 2016. Web. <davesgarden.com/guides/articles/view/2492/>
3. Harrison, Marie. "Blue-eyed Grass." *Dave's Garden,* January 6, 2016. Web. <davesgarden.com/guides/articles/view/2492/>
4. Harrison, Marie. "Blue-eyed Grass." *Dave's Garden,* January 6, 2016. Web. <davesgarden.com/guides/articles/view/2492/>
5. "Sisyrinchium angustifolium." *Lady Bird Johnson Wildflower Center Plant Database,* April 1, 2017. Web. <http://www.wildflower.org/plants/result.php?id_plant=sian3>
6. "Sisyrinchium bellum." *Wikipedia: The Free Encyclopedia,* August 8, 2016. Web. <en.wikipedia.org/wiki/Sisyrinchium_bellum>
7. "The Presidio of San Francisco: Blue-eyed Grass (Sisyrinchium bellum)." *National Park Service,* August 8, 2016. Web. <nps.gov/prsf/learn/nature/blue-eyed-grass.htm>
8. "Blue-eyed Grass – Sisyrinchium angustifolium." *Herbe Rowe,* January 6, 2016. Web. <herberowe.wordpress.com/2011/05/27/blue-eyed-grass-sisyrinchium-angustifolium/>
10. "Mountain Blue-eyed Grass." January 6, 2016. Web. <montana.plant-life.org/species/sisyr_monta.htm>
11. "The Presidio of San Francisco: Blue-eyed Grass (Sisyrinchium bellum)." *National Park Service,* August 8, 2016. Web. <nps.gov/prsf/learn/nature/blue-eyed-grass.htm>
12. "Mountain Blue-eyed Grass." January 6, 2016. Web. <montana.plant-life.org/species/sisyr_monta.htm>
13. Harrison, Marie. "Blue-eyed Grass." *Dave's Garden,* January 6, 2016. Web. <davesgarden.com/guides/articles/view/2492/>
14. "Sisyrinchium bellum." *Wikipedia: The Free Encyclopedia,* August 8, 2016. Web. <en.wikipedia.org/wiki/Sisyrinchium_bellum>
15. Harrison, Marie. "Blue-eyed Grass." *Dave's Garden,* January 6, 2016. Web. <davesgarden.com/guides/articles/view/2492/>
16. "Blue-eyed Grass – Sisyrinchium angustifolium." *Herbe Rowe,* January 6, 2016. Web. <herberowe.wordpress.com/2011/05/27/blue-eyed-grass-sisyrinchium-angustifolium/>

BLUE GUM EUCALYPTUS

1. "Eucalyptus globulus." *Wikipedia: The Free Encyclopedia,* August 8, 2016. Web. <Wikipedia.org/wiki/Eucalyptus_globulus>
2. "Medicinal Uses & Benefits of Eucalyptus." *Annie's Remedy: Essential Oils and Herbs,* August 10, 2016. Web. <anniesremedy.com /herb_detail23.php>
3. "Find a Vitamin or Supplement: EUCALYPTUS." *WebMD,* August 10, 2016. Web. <http://www.webmd.com/vitamins-supplements/ingredientmono-700-eucalyptus.aspx?activeingredientid=700&activeingredientname=eucalyptus>
4. Skenderi, Gazmend. "Eucalyptus." *Herbal Vade Mecum.* Rutherford, New Jersey: Herbacy Press, 2003. Print.
5. Skenderi, Gazmend. "Eucalyptus." *Herbal Vade Mecum.* Rutherford, New Jersey: Herbacy Press, 2003. Print.
6. "Find a Vitamin or Supplement: EUCALYPTUS." *WebMD,* August 10, 2016. Web. <http://www.webmd.com/vitamins-supplements/ingredientmono-700-eucalyptus.aspx?activeingredientid=700&activeingredientname=eucalyptus>
7. Skenderi, Gazmend. "Eucalyptus." *Herbal Vade Mecum.* Rutherford, New Jersey: Herbacy Press, 2003. Print.
8. "About Eucalyptus globulus and 1,8 cineole." *The School For Aromatic Studies,* August 12, 2016. Web. < http://theida.com/about-eucalyptus-globulus-and-18-cineole>
9. "Find a Vitamin or Supplement: EUCALYPTUS." *WebMD,* August 10, 2016. Web. <http://www.webmd.com/vitamins-supplements/ingredientmono-700-eucalyptus.aspx?activeingredientid=700&activeingredientname=eucalyptus>
10. "Find a Vitamin or Supplement: EUCALYPTUS." *WebMD,* August 10, 2016. Web. <http://www.webmd.com/vitamins-supplements/ingredientmono-700-eucalyptus.aspx?activeingredientid=700&activeingredientname=eucalyptus>
11. Skenderi, Gazmend. "Eucalyptus." *Herbal Vade Mecum.* Rutherford, New Jersey: Herbacy Press, 2003. Print.
12. "Medicinal Uses & Benefits of Eucalyptus." *Annie's Remedy: Essential Oils and Herbs,* August 10, 2016. Web. <anniesremedy.com /herb_detail23.php>
13. "About Eucalyptus globulus and 1,8 cineole." *The School For Aromatic Studies,* August 12, 2016. Web. < http://theida.com/about-eucalyptus-globulus-and-18-cineole>
14. "Medicinal Uses & Benefits of Eucalyptus." *Annie's Remedy: Essential Oils and Herbs,* August 10, 2016. Web. <anniesremedy.com /herb_detail23.php>

15. "Eucalyptus Oil: Essential Oil Extraordinaire." *Mercola.com: Take Control of Your Health,* August 10, 2016. Web. <articles.mercola.com/herbal-oils/eucalyptus-oil.aspx>
16. Skenderi, Gazmend. "Eucalyptus." *Herbal Vade Mecum.* Rutherford, New Jersey: Herbacy Press, 2003. Print.
17. "Eucalyptus Oil: Essential Oil Extraordinaire." *Mercola.com: Take Control of Your Health,* August 10, 2016. Web. <articles.mercola.com/herbal-oils/eucalyptus-oil.aspx>
18. "Medicinal Uses & Benefits of Eucalyptus." *Annie's Remedy: Essential Oils and Herbs,* August 10, 2016. Web. <anniesremedy.com /herb_detail23.php>
19. Rowland, Teisha. "How the Eucalyptus Came to California: A Cautionary Tale," *Santa Barbara Independent,* January 15, 2011. Web. <independent.com/news/2011/jan/15/how-eucalyptus-came-california>
20. "Find a Vitamin or Supplement: EUCALYPTUS." *WebMD,* August 10, 2016. Web. <http://www.webmd.com/vitamins-supplements/ingredientmono-700-eucalyptus.aspx?activeingredientid=700&activeingredientname=eucalyptus>
21. Rowland, Teisha. "How the Eucalyptus Came to California: A Cautionary Tale," *Santa Barbara Independent,* January 15, 2011. Web. <independent.com/news/2011/jan/15/how-eucalyptus-came-california>
22. Rowland, Teisha. "How the Eucalyptus Came to California: A Cautionary Tale," *Santa Barbara Independent,* January 15, 2011. Web. <independent.com/news/2011/jan/15/how-eucalyptus-came-california>
23. Rowland, Teisha. "How the Eucalyptus Came to California: A Cautionary Tale," *Santa Barbara Independent,* January 15, 2011. Web. <independent.com/news/2011/jan/15/how-eucalyptus-came-california>
24. "Eucalyptus globulus." *Wikipedia: The Free Encyclopedia,* August 8, 2016. Web. <Wikipedia.org/wiki/Eucalyptus_globulus>
25. Rowland, Teisha. "How the Eucalyptus Came to California: A Cautionary Tale," *Santa Barbara Independent,* January 15, 2011. Web. <independent.com/news/2011/jan/15/how-eucalyptus-came-california>

CALENDULA

1. Johnson, Rebecca, et al. *National Geographic Guide to Medicinal Herbs: The World's Most Effective Healing Plants.* Washington DC: National Geographic Society, 2012. Print.
2. Johnson, Rebecca, et al. *National Geographic Guide to Medicinal Herbs: The World's Most Effective Healing Plants.* Washington DC: National Geographic Society, 2012. Print.
3. "Benefits of Calendula." Healing from Home Remedies, October 1, 2016. Web. <www.healing-from-home-remedies.com/benefits-of-calendula.html>
4. Skenderi, Gazmend. "Calendula." *Herbal Vade Mecum.* Rutherford, New Jersey: Herbacy Press, 2003. Print.
5. Skenderi, Gazmend. "Calendula." *Herbal Vade Mecum.* Rutherford, New Jersey: Herbacy Press, 2003. Print.
6. "Benefits of Calendula." Healing from Home Remedies, October 1, 2016. Web. <www.healing-from-home-remedies.com/benefits-of-calendula.html>
7. Skenderi, Gazmend. "Calendula." *Herbal Vade Mecum.* Rutherford, New Jersey: Herbacy Press, 2003. Print.
8. Herbal Academy of New England: The Online Intermediate Herbal Course, October 1, 2016 <http://members.herbalacademyofne.com/course/intermediate-herbal-course>
9. Skenderi, Gazmend. "Calendula." *Herbal Vade Mecum.* Rutherford, New Jersey: Herbacy Press, 2003. Print.
10. Benefits of Calendula." Healing from Home Remedies, October 1, 2016. Web. <www.healing-from-home-remedies.com/benefits-of-calendula.html>
11. Johnson, Rebecca, et al. *National Geographic Guide to Medicinal Herbs: The World's Most Effective Healing Plants.* Washington DC: National Geographic Society, 2012. Print.
12. Benefits of Calendula." Healing from Home Remedies, October 1, 2016. Web. <www.healing-from-home-remedies.com/benefits-of-calendula.html>
13. Skenderi, Gazmend. "Calendula." *Herbal Vade Mecum.* Rutherford, New Jersey: Herbacy Press, 2003. Print.
14. Benefits of Calendula." Healing from Home Remedies, October 1, 2016. Web. <www.healing-from-home-remedies.com/benefits-of-calendula.html>
15. Benefits of Calendula." Healing from Home Remedies, October 1, 2016. Web. <www.healing-from-home-remedies.com/benefits-of-calendula.html>
16. Johnson, Rebecca, et al. *National Geographic Guide to Medicinal Herbs: The World's Most Effective Healing Plants.* Washington DC: National Geographic Society, 2012. Print.
17. "Calendula." Wikipedia: The Free Encyclopedia, September 10, 2016. Web. <https://en.wikipedia.org/wiki/Calendula>
18. Johnson, Rebecca, et al. *National Geographic Guide to Medicinal Herbs: The World's Most Effective Healing Plants.* Washington DC: National Geographic Society, 2012. Print.
19. Johnson, Rebecca, et al. *National Geographic Guide to Medicinal Herbs: The World's Most Effective Healing Plants.* Washington DC: National Geographic Society, 2012. Print.
20. "Calendula." Herbal Encyclopedia: Common medicinal herbs for natural health, September 13, 2016. Web. <http://www.cloverleaffarmherbs.com/calendula>

1. "Calendula." Wikipedia: The Free Encyclopedia, September 10, 2016. Web. <https://en.wikipedia.org/wiki/Calendula>
22. "Calendula." Herbal Encyclopedia: Common medicinal herbs for natural health, September 13, 2016. Web. <http://www.cloverleaffarmherbs.com/calendula>
23. "Calendula." Herbal Encyclopedia: Common medicinal herbs for natural health, September 13, 2016. Web. <http://www.cloverleaffarmherbs.com/calendula>
24. "Calendula." Herbal Encyclopedia: Common medicinal herbs for natural health, September 13, 2016. Web. <http://www.cloverleaffarmherbs.com/calendula>
25. "Calendula." Wikipedia: The Free Encyclopedia, September 10, 2016. Web. <https://en.wikipedia.org/wiki/Calendula>
26. "Calendula." Herbal Encyclopedia: Common medicinal herbs for natural health, September 13, 2016. Web. <http://www.cloverleaffarmherbs.com/calendula>
27. "About Calendula." Gardenguides.com, July 3, 2015. Web. <www.gardenguides.com/69834-calendula.html>
28. "About Calendula." Gardenguides.com, July 3, 2015. Web. <www.gardenguides.com/69834-calendula.html>
29. "Calendula." Herbal Encyclopedia: Common medicinal herbs for natural health, September 13, 2016. Web. <http://www.cloverleaffarmherbs.com/calendula>
30. Wikipedia, "Calendula." Web. <https://en.wikipedia.org/wiki/Calendula> September 10, 2016
31. "About Calendula." Gardenguides.com, July 3, 2015. Web. <www.gardenguides.com/69834-calendula.html>
32. "Calendula." Herbal Encyclopedia: Common medicinal herbs for natural health, September 13, 2016. Web. <http://www.cloverleaffarmherbs.com/calendula>
33. "About Calendula." Gardenguides.com, July 3, 2015. Web. <www.gardenguides.com/69834-calendula.html>
34. "Why not plant some Calendula?" Root Simple: low tech home tech, September 10, 2016. Web. <http://www.rootsimple.com/2011/02/why-not-plant-some-calendula>
35. "Why not plant some Calendula?" Root Simple: low tech home tech, September 10, 2016. Web. <http://www.rootsimple.com/2011/02/why-not-plant-some-calendula>

OTHER SOURCES:

"Harvesting and Drying Calendula." *Root Simple: low tech home tech,* September 10, 2016. Web. < rootsimple.com/2011/03/harvesting-and-drying-calendula>
"How to make a Calendula oil infusion." *Root Simple: low tech home tech,* September 10, 2016. Web. < rootsimple.com/2011/07/how-to-make-a-calendula-oil-infusion >
"Calendula officinalis • Zergul • Marigold." *Anne Mcuntyre: Herbal Medicine Ayurvada,* October 3, 2016. Web. <http://annemcintyre.com/calendula-officinalis-%E2%80%A2-zergul-%E2%80%A2-marigold>
"Calendula Flowers." *Mountain rose herbs.com,* October 1, 2016. Web. <https://www.mountainroseherbs.com/products/calendula-flowers/profile>

CALIFORNIA BAY

1. Moore, Michael. "California Bay." *Medicinal Plants of the Pacific West.* Santa Fe, NM: Red Crane Books, 1993. Print.
2. Moore, Michael. "California Bay." *Medicinal Plants of the Pacific West.* Santa Fe, NM: Red Crane Books, 1993. Print.
3. "Bay leaf nutrition facts." *www.nutrition-and-you.com,* October 17, 2016. <http://www.nutrition-and-you.com/bay-leaf.html>
4. "Bay leaf nutrition facts." *www.nutrition-and-you.com,* October 17, 2016. <http://www.nutrition-and-you.com/bay-leaf.html>
5. Moore, Michael. "California Bay." *Medicinal Plants of the Pacific West.* Santa Fe, NM: Red Crane Books, 1993. Print.
6. "Bay leaf nutrition facts." *www.nutrition-and-you.com,* October 17, 2016. <http://www.nutrition-and-you.com/bay-leaf.html>
7. "Bay leaf nutrition facts." *www.nutrition-and-you.com,* October 17, 2016. <http://www.nutrition-and-you.com/bay-leaf.html>
8. "Bay leaf nutrition facts." *www.nutrition-and-you.com,* October 17, 2016. <http://www.nutrition-and-you.com/bay-leaf.html>
9. Moore, Michael. "California Bay." *Medicinal Plants of the Pacific West.* Santa Fe, NM: Red Crane Books, 1993. Print.
10. Moore, Michael. "California Bay." *Medicinal Plants of the Pacific West.* Santa Fe, NM: Red Crane Books, 1993. Print.
11. Moore, Michael. "California Bay." *Medicinal Plants of the Pacific West.* Santa Fe, NM: Red Crane Books, 1993. Print.
12. Moore, Michael. "California Bay." *Medicinal Plants of the Pacific West.* Santa Fe, NM: Red Crane Books, 1993. Print.

13. Moore, Michael. "California Bay." *Medicinal Plants of the Pacific West*. Santa Fe, NM: Red Crane Books, 1993. Print.
14. Moore, Michael. "California Bay." *Medicinal Plants of the Pacific West*. Santa Fe, NM: Red Crane Books, 1993. Print.
15. "Bay leaf nutrition facts." *www.nutrition-and-you.com,* October 17, 2016. <http://www.nutrition-and-you.com/bay-leaf.html>
16. "Bay leaf nutrition facts." *www.nutrition-and-you.com,* October 17, 2016. <http://www.nutrition-and-you.com/bay-leaf.html>
17. Moore, Michael. "California Bay." *Medicinal Plants of the Pacific West*. Santa Fe, NM: Red Crane Books, 1993. Print.
18. "Medicinal herbs, California Laurel, Umbellularia californica." *Herbs,* July 25, 2015. <http://naturalmedicinalherbs.net/herbs/u/umbellularia-californica=california-laurel.php>
19. "Apollo and Daphne." *Greeka.com: The Greek Island Specialist,* October 11, 2016. <http://www.greeka.com/greece-myths/apollo-daphne.htm>
20. "Apollo and Daphne." *Greeka.com: The Greek Island Specialist,* October 11, 2016. <http://www.greeka.com/greece-myths/apollo-daphne.htm>
21. "Apollo and Daphne." *Wikipedia: The Free Encyclopedia,* July 25, 2016. <https://en.wikipedia.org/wiki/Apollo_and_Daphne>
22. "17 AMAZING Bay Laurel Essential Oil Uses and Benefits That Will Surprise You." *Essential Oils informer,* October 17, 2016. < http://essentialoilsinformer.com/17-amazing-bay-laurel-essential-oil-uses-and-benefits-that-will-surprise-you>
23. "Bay leaf nutrition facts." *www.nutrition-and-you.com,* October 17, 2016. <http://www.nutrition-and-you.com/bay-leaf.html>
24. "17 AMAZING Bay Laurel Essential Oil Uses and Benefits That Will Surprise You." *Essential Oils informer,* October 17, 2016. <http://essentialoilsinformer.com/17-amazing-bay-laurel-essential-oil-uses-and-benefits-that-will-surprise-you>
25. "Apollo and Daphne." *Wikipedia: The Free Encyclopedia,* July 25, 2016 <https://en.wikipedia.org/wiki/Apollo_and_Daphne>
26. "Umbellularia Californica (Hook. And Arn.) Nutt-California bay tree; California olive-Lauraceae." <http://www.botanicalbeads.com/BBB_page_15.html> July 25, 2015
27. "Umbellularia Californica (Hook. And Arn.) Nutt-California bay tree; California olive-Lauraceae." July 25, 2015. <http://www.botanicalbeads.com/BBB_page_15.html>
28. "Bay leaf nutrition facts." *www.nutrition-and-you.com,* October 17, 2016. <http://www.nutrition-and-you.com/bay-leaf.html>
29. Moore, Michael. "California Bay." *Medicinal Plants of the Pacific West*. Santa Fe, NM: Red Crane Books, 1993. Print.
30. Moore, Michael. "California Bay." *Medicinal Plants of the Pacific West*. Santa Fe, NM: Red Crane Books, 1993. Print.
31. "Bay leaf nutrition facts." *www.nutrition-and-you.com,* October 17, 2016. <http://www.nutrition-and-you.com/bay-leaf.html>

CALIFORNIA POPPY

1. Moore, Michael. "California Poppy." *Medicinal Plants of the Pacific West*. Santa Fe, NM: Red Crane Books, 1993. Print.
2. "California Poppy, Eschscholzia californica." *Annies Remedy: Essential Oils and Herbs,* January 9, 2016. Web. <https://www.anniesremedy.com/eschscholzia-californica-poppy.php>
3. "California Poppy, Eschscholzia californica." *Annies Remedy: Essential Oils and Herbs,* January 9, 2016. Web. <https://www.anniesremedy.com/eschscholzia-californica-poppy.php>
4. "California Poppy, Eschscholzia californica." *Annies Remedy: Essential Oils and Herbs,* January 9, 2016. Web. <https://www.anniesremedy.com/eschscholzia-californica-poppy.php>
5. "California Poppy." *Smokable Herbs,* January 19, 2012. Web. <smokableherbs.com/California-poppy/# History-and-Use>
6. Moore, Michael. "California Poppy." *Medicinal Plants of the Pacific West*. Santa Fe, NM: Red Crane Books, 1993. Print.
7. Moore, Michael. "California Poppy." *Medicinal Plants of the Pacific West*. Santa Fe, NM: Red Crane Books, 1993. Print.
8. Katz, Richard and Patricia Kaminski. "California Poppy Profile: True Gold is in the Heart." *Flower essence society,* December 20, 2016. Web. <http://www.flowersociety.org/california-poppy.html>
9. Katz, Richard and Patricia Kaminski. "California Poppy Profile: True Gold is in the Heart." *Flower essence society,* December 20, 2016. Web. <http://www.flowersociety.org/california-poppy.html>
10. Katz, Richard and Patricia Kaminski. "California Poppy Profile: True Gold is in the Heart." *Flower essence society,* December 20, 2016. Web. <http://www.flowersociety.org/california-poppy.html>
11. Katz, Richard and Patricia Kaminski. "California Poppy Profile: True Gold is in the Heart." *Flower essence society,* December 20, 2016. Web. <http://www.flowersociety.org/california-poppy.html>

2. "California Poppy." *Smokable Herbs,* January 19, 2012. Web. <smokableherbs.com/California-poppy/# History-and-Use>

OTHER SOURCES:

"Monterey Bay Spice Company_ Eschscholzia californica California Poppy Plant overview beauty and the California Poppy." January 9, 2016. Web. <herb.co.com?c-213-california-poppy.aspx>

"Sleep Disorders Advise & Help." November 6, 2016. Web. <http://sleepdisorders.dolyan.com/health-benefits-of-california-poppy>

"California Poppy." Medical Medium Blog, November 6, 2016. Web. < http://www.medicalmedium.com/blog/california-poppy>

CALIFORNIA TIGER LILY

1. Tiger Lily Benefits-Lilium Lancifolium Uses and Side Effects." *In 4 Nation Health,* July 27, 2016. Web. <health.in4nation.com/tiger-lily-benefits-lilium-lancifolium-use>
2. "Tiger Lily Benefits-Lilium Lancifolium Uses and Side Effects." *In 4 Nation Health,* July 27, 2016. Web. <health.in4nation.com/tiger-lily-benefits-lilium-lancifolium-use>
3. "Tiger Lily Lilium lancifolium." *Herbs,* March 20, 2017. Web. <naturalmedicinalherbs.net/herbs/l/lilium-lancifolium=tiger-lily.php>
4. "Tiger Lily Benefits-Lilium Lancifolium Uses and Side Effects." *In 4 Nation Health,* July 27, 2016. Web. <health.in4nation.com/tiger-lily-benefits-lilium-lancifolium-use>
5. "Tiger Lily Benefits-Lilium Lancifolium Uses and Side Effects." *In 4 Nation Health,* July 27, 2016. Web. <health.in4nation.com/tiger-lily-benefits-lilium-lancifolium-use>
6. "Tiger Lily Benefits-Lilium Lancifolium Uses and Side Effects." *In 4 Nation Health,* July 27, 2016. Web. <health.in4nation.com/tiger-lily-benefits-lilium-lancifolium-use>
7. "Tiger Lily Benefits-Lilium Lancifolium Uses and Side Effects." *In 4 Nation Health,* July 27, 2016. Web. <health.in4nation.com/tiger-lily-benefits-lilium-lancifolium-use>
8. "Tiger Lily." *Pet Poison Helpline,* May 26, 2017. Web. <petpoisonhelpline.com/poison/tiger-lily/>
9. "Lilium pardalinum." *Revolvy,* March 20, 2017. Web. <https://www.revolvy.com/main/index.php?s=Lilium%20pardalinum>
10. Lyons, Kathleen and Mary Beth Cooney-Lazaneo. "Blue Elderberry," *Plants of the Coast Redwood Region.* Boulder Creek, CA. Looking Press, 1988. Print.
11. About Tiger Lillies, *Tiger Lily,* March 20, 2017. Web. <tigerlilyflower.blogspot.com>
12. "Lilium pardalinum (Leopard Lily, California Tiger Lily)." *Golden Gate National Parks Conservancy,* July 27, 2016. Web. <parksconservancy.org/conservation/plants-animals/native-plant-information/california-tiger-lilly.html>
13. "Tiger Lily Benefits-Lilium Lancifolium Uses and Side Effects." *In 4 Nation Health,* July 27, 2016. Web. <health.in4nation.com/tiger-lily-benefits-lilium-lancifolium-use>
14. "Tiger Lily Benefits-Lilium Lancifolium Uses and Side Effects." *In 4 Nation Health,* July 27, 2016. Web. <health.in4nation.com/tiger-lily-benefits-lilium-lancifolium-use>
15. "Lilium pardalinum." *Revolvy,* March 20, 2017. Web. <https://www.revolvy.com/main/index.php?s=Lilium%20pardalinum>

OTHER SOURCES:

"The flower expert Tiger Lily." *Gifting inc,* July 27, 2016. Web. <theflowerexpert.com/content/aboutflowers/tiger-lily>

Carter, Karen. "Facts About the Tiger Lily Flower." July 27, 2016. Web. <homeguides.com/Tiger-lily-flower-48318.html>

COTTONWOOD

1. "Benefits and Use of Balm of Gilead with Herbalist Yarrow Willard | Harmonic Arts." *Harmonic Arts Botanical Dispensary*, December 22, 2016. Web. <https://www.youtube.com/watch?v=uPEpIcGn1OI>
2. "How to Make Cottonwood Salve." *Alderleaf Wilderness College,* December 22, 2016. Web. <http://www.wildernesscollege.com/cottonwood-salve.html>
3. "How to Make Cottonwood Salve." *Alderleaf Wilderness College,* December 22, 2016. Web. <http://www.wildernesscollege.com/cottonwood-salve.html>
4. "How to Make Cottonwood Salve." *Alderleaf Wilderness College,* December 22, 2016. Web. <http://www.wildernesscollege.com/cottonwood-salve.html>
5. "Benefits and Use of Balm of Gilead with Herbalist Yarrow Willard | Harmonic Arts." *Harmonic Arts Botanical Dispensary*, December 22, 2016. Web. <https://www.youtube.com/watch?v=uPEpIcGn1OI>
6. "Benefits and Use of Balm of Gilead with Herbalist Yarrow Willard | Harmonic Arts." *Harmonic Arts Botanical Dispensary*, December 22, 2016. Web. <https://www.youtube.com/watch?v=uPEpIcGn1OI>
7. "Benefits and Use of Balm of Gilead with Herbalist Yarrow Willard | Harmonic Arts." *Harmonic Arts Botanical Dispensary*, December 22, 2016. Web. <https://www.youtube.com/watch?v=uPEpIcGn1OI>

8.   "Benefits and Use of Balm of Gilead with Herbalist Yarrow Willard | Harmonic Arts." *Harmonic Arts Botanical Dispensary*, December 22, 2016. Web. <https://www.youtube.com/watch?v=uPEpIcGn1OI>
OTHER SOURCES:
Wild Foods & Medicines, "Cottonwood Bud." <http://wildfoodsandmedicines.com/test-post> December 22, 2016.

DANDELION

1.   "Here are some interesting facts about the dandelion flower." *My dandelion is a flower,* December 24, 2016. Web. <http://mydandelionisaflower.org/did-you-know>
2.   "Dandelion overview." *University of Maryland Medical Center,* June 11, 2016. Web. <umm.edu/health/medical/altmed/herb/dandelion>
3.   Skenderi, Gazmend. "Dandelion." *Herbal Vade Mecum.* Rutherford, New Jersey: Herbacy Press, 2003. Print.
4.   "Dandelion overview." *University of Maryland Medical Center,* June 11, 2016. Web. <umm.edu/health/medical/altmed/herb/dandelion>
5.   "Dandelion overview." *University of Maryland Medical Center,* June 11, 2016. Web. <umm.edu/health/medical/altmed/herb/dandelion>
6.   "Dandelion overview." *University of Maryland Medical Center,* June 11, 2016. Web. <umm.edu/health/medical/altmed/herb/dandelion>
7.   "Health Benefits of Dandelion." *Organic Facts,* June 11, 2016. Web. <organicfacts.net/health-benefits/herbs-and-spices/health-benefits-of-dandelion.html>
8.   "Dandelion Salve Recipe." *The Nerdy Farm Wife,* June 14, 2016. <https://thenerdyfarmwife.com/dandelion-salve-recipe>
9.   "Dandelion overview." *University of Maryland Medical Center,* June 11, 2016. Web. <umm.edu/health/medical/altmed/herb/dandelion>
10.   "Making and Using Dandelion Oil." *Homespun Seasonal Living: cultivating a courageous and fiercely D.I.Y. lifestyle,* June 11, 2016. Web. <homespunseasonalliving.com/making-and-using-dandelion-oil>
11.   "Dandelion overview." *University of Maryland Medical Center,* June 11, 2016. Web. <umm.edu/health/medical/altmed/herb/dandelion>
12.   Skenderi, Gazmend. "Dandelion." *Herbal Vade Mecum.* Rutherford, New Jersey: Herbacy Press, 2003. Print.
13.   "Dandelion overview." *University of Maryland Medical Center,* June 11, 2016. Web. <umm.edu/health/medical/altmed/herb/dandelion>
14.   "Dandelion Myths, Legends, and Folklore." *CHANGINGLIFESTYLEBLOG,* June 11, 2016. Web. < https://changinglifestyleblog.wordpress.com/2011/04/12/dandelion-myths-legends-and-folklore>
15.   "Dandelion Myths, Legends, and Folklore." *CHANGINGLIFESTYLEBLOG,* June 11, 2016. Web. < https://changinglifestyleblog.wordpress.com/2011/04/12/dandelion-myths-legends-and-folklore>
16.   "Dandelion Myths, Legends, and Folklore." *CHANGINGLIFESTYLEBLOG,* June 11, 2016. Web. < https://changinglifestyleblog.wordpress.com/2011/04/12/dandelion-myths-legends-and-folklore>
OTHER SOURCES:
"Health Benefits of Dandelion." *Organic Facts,* June 11, 2016. Web. <organicfacts.net/health-benefits/herbs-and-spices/health-benefits-of-dandelion.html>
Grieve, Mrs. M. "Dandelion." *Botanical.com,* June 11, 2016. Web. <botanical.com/botanical/nigmh/d/dandel08.html>
"Dandelion Herb Uses, Health Benefits, and Side Effects." *Medical Health Guide: Blending Natural & Modern Medicine,* June 11, 2016. Web. <Medicalhealthguide.com/herb/dandelion.com.html>
"Dandelion Magnesium Lotion." *The Nerdy Farm Wife,* June 11, 2016. Web. <thenerdyfarmwife.com/dandelion-magnesium-lotion>

FALSE SOLOMON'S SEAL

1.   Thayer, Samuel. "False Solomon's Seal, Solomon's Plume." *Nature's Garden: A Guide to Identifying, Harvesting, and Preparing Edible Wild Plants,* (Birchwood, WI: Forager's Harvest Press, 2010), 91-98.
2.   Thayer, Samuel. "False Solomon's Seal, Solomon's Plume." *Nature's Garden: A Guide to Identifying, Harvesting, and Preparing Edible Wild Plants,* (Birchwood, WI: Forager's Harvest Press, 2010), 91-98.
3.   Moore, Michael. "False Solomon's Seal," *Medicinal Plants of the Pacific West,* (Santa Fe, NM: Red Crane Books, 1993), 131-133.
4.   *Wild Edible and Medicinal Plants~using what nature provides in plants,* "Wild Edible and Medicinal Plants 113-114 False Solomon's Seal/Nut Grass." December 28, 2016. <https://keys2liberty.wordpress.com//?s=False+Solomon%27s+Seal&search=Go>
5.   Medicine club
6.   Moore, Michael. "False Solomon's Seal," *Medicinal Plants of the Pacific West,* (Santa Fe, NM: Red Crane Books, 1993), 131-133.

. *Wild Edible and Medicinal Plants~using what nature provides in plants,* "Wild Edible and Medicinal Plants 113-114 False Solomon's Seal/Nut Grass." December 28, 2016. <https://keys2liberty.wordpress.com//?s=False+Solomon%27s+Seal&search=Go>

. Moore, Michael. "False Solomon's Seal," *Medicinal Plants of the Pacific West,* (Santa Fe, NM: Red Crane Books, 1993), 131-133.

). Moore, Michael. "False Solomon's Seal," *Medicinal Plants of the Pacific West,* (Santa Fe, NM: Red Crane Books, 1993), 131-133.

10. *Wild Edible and Medicinal Plants~using what nature provides in plants,* "Wild Edible and Medicinal Plants 113-114 False Solomon's Seal/Nut Grass." December 28, 2016. <https://keys2liberty.wordpress.com//?s=False+Solomon%27s+Seal&search=Go>

11. Moore, Michael. "False Solomon's Seal," *Medicinal Plants of the Pacific West,* (Santa Fe, NM: Red Crane Books, 1993), 131-133.

12. Thayer, Samuel. "False Solomon's Seal, Solomon's Plume." *Nature's Garden: A Guide to Identifying, Harvesting, and Preparing Edible Wild Plants,* (Birchwood, WI: Forager's Harvest Press, 2010), 91-98.

13. Thayer, Samuel. "False Solomon's Seal, Solomon's Plume." *Nature's Garden: A Guide to Identifying, Harvesting, and Preparing Edible Wild Plants,* (Birchwood, WI: Forager's Harvest Press, 2010), 91-98.

14. Go Wild Institute, Awaken Your Nature. "False Solomon's Seal Journey: from the magician to the dragon." December 29, 2016. Web. <http://myemail.constantcontact.com/Awaken-Your-Nature-.html?soid=1103157481513&aid=BUhrCmZPXxA>

15. Vizgirdas, Ray S. and Edna M. Rey-Vizgirdas. December 28, 2016. "Wild Plants of the Sierra Nevada." Web. <https://books.google.com/books?id=2LB4OQLv-w8C&pg=PA230&lpg=PA230&dq=false+solomon's+seal+kidney&source=bl&ots=5B7CNftXf_&sig=ZS0L53> Page 230.

OTHER SOURCES
The Medicine Club, "False Solomon's Seal." December 28, 2016.
<http://themedicineclub.blogspot.com/2008/09/this-weeks-plant-was-false-solomons.html>

FENNEL

1. "Fennel:Administration and Indications Guide,Dosages and Safety." *M Didea,* August 6, 2015. Web. <https://www.mdidea.com/products/new/new04205.html>

2. "Fennel (Foeniculum vulgare)." *Herbwisdom.com, the number 1 source of herb information,* December 22, 2016. Web. <http://www.herbwisdom.com/herb-fennel.html>

3. "Fennel (Foeniculum vulgare)." *Herbwisdom.com, the number 1 source of herb information,* December 22, 2016. Web. <http://www.herbwisdom.com/herb-fennel.html>

4. "Fennel (Foeniculum vulgare)." *Herbwisdom.com, the number 1 source of herb information,* December 22, 2016. Web. <http://www.herbwisdom.com/herb-fennel.html>

5. "Fennel (Foeniculum vulgare)." *Herbwisdom.com, the number 1 source of herb information,* December 22, 2016. Web. <http://www.herbwisdom.com/herb-fennel.html>

6. "Fennel:Administration and Indications Guide,Dosages and Safety." *M Didea,* August 6, 2015. Web. <https://www.mdidea.com/products/new/new04205.html>

7. Johnson, Rebecca L, et al. National *Geographic Guide to Medicinal Herbs: The World's Most Effective Healing Plants.* Washington DC, USA: National Geographic Society, 2012. Print.

8. Gioia, Maria. "Fennel and Miscarriage." *Natural Health for Fertility and Pregnancy,* March 21, 2017. Web. <natural-health-for-fertility.com/fennel-and-miscarriage.html>

9. "Fennel:Administration and Indications Guide,Dosages and Safety." *M Didea,* August 6, 2015. Web. <https://www.mdidea.com/products/new/new04205.html>

10. Kirkpatrick, Naida. "The Sumarians." Chacago, Il: Heinmann Library, 2003. Print.

11. "Fennel Legends, Myths, and Stories." *M Didea,* August 6, 2015. Web. <https://www.mdidea.com/products/new/new04205.html>

12. Johnson, Rebecca L, et al. National *Geographic Guide to Medicinal Herbs: The World's Most Effective Healing Plants.* Washington DC, USA: National Geographic Society, 2012. Print.

13. "Fennel Legends, Myths, and Stories." *Didea,* August 6, 2015. Web. <https://www.mdidea.com/products/new/new04205.html>

GIANT KELP

1. Medical Herb Info. "Kelp." May 31, 2016. Web. <medicalherbinfo.org/herbs/kelp.html>
2. Medical Herb Info. "Kelp." May 31, 2016. Web. <medicalherbinfo.org/herbs/kelp.html>
3. Medical Herb Info. "Kelp." May 31, 2016. Web. <medicalherbinfo.org/herbs/kelp.html>
4. Medical Herb Info, "Kelp." May 31, 2016. Web. <medicalherbinfo.org/herbs/kelp.html>
5. Drum, Ryan. "Sea Vegetables For Food and Medicine." May 31, 2016. Web

6.   Medical Herb Info. "Kelp." May 31, 2016. Web. <medicalherbinfo.org/herbs/kelp.html>
7.   Drum, Ryan. "Sea Vegetables For Food and Medicine." May 31, 2016. Web. <ryandrum.com/expan1.html>
8.   Medical Health Guide. "Kelp Health Benefits." May 31, 2016. Web. <medicalhealthguide.com/articles/kelp.htm>
9.   Medical Herb Info. "Kelp." May 31, 2016. Web. <medicalherbinfo.org/herbs/kelp.html>
10.   Drum, Ryan. "Sea Vegetables For Food and Medicine." May 31, 2016. Web. <ryandrum.com/expan1.html>
11.   Medical Herb Info. "Kelp." May 31, 2016. Web. <medicalherbinfo.org/herbs/kelp.html>

OTHER SOURCES:

FAO corporate document repository. "Descriptions and uses of plant foods by Indigenous Peoples: Algae (Seaweeds)." May 31, 2016. Web. <fao.org/wairdocs/other/ai/5e/A1215E06.htm>

University of Southern California Sea Giant Program. "Help With Kelp." May 31, 2016. Web. <dornsite.UCSC.edu/assets/sites/291/docs/kelp-Handout.pdf>

AIHDP. "Foods Indigenous to the Western Hemisphere: Giant Kelp." May 31, 2016. Web. <web.ku.edu/~aihd/foods/giant_kelp.html>

HIMALAYAN BLACKBERRY

1.   Falconi, Dina. *Earthly Bodies & Heavenly Hair.* Woodstock, NY:Ceres Press, 1998
2.   Jackson, Deb, and Karen Bergeron. Alternative Nature Online Herbal. "Blackberry Edible, Herbal use and Medicinal Properties." June 14, 2016. Web. <https://altnature.com/gallery/blackberry.htm>
3.   Chickadee Apothecary. "Bramble On, Blackberry: Wild Food & Medicine." June 14, 2016. Web. <https://www.chickadeeapothecary.com/blogs/chickadee-apothecary/14660107-bramble-on-blackberry-wild-food-medicine>
4.   Chickadee Apothecary. "Bramble On, Blackberry: Wild Food & Medicine." June 14, 2016. Web. <https://www.chickadeeapothecary.com/blogs/chickadee-apothecary/14660107-bramble-on-blackberry-wild-food-medicine>
5.   Jackson, Deb, and Karen Bergeron. Alternative Nature Online Herbal. "Blackberry Edible, Herbal use and Medicinal Properties." June 14, 2016. Web. <https://altnature.com/gallery/blackberry.htm>
6.   Chickadee Apothecary. "Bramble On, Blackberry: Wild Food & Medicine." June 14, 2016. Web. <https://www.chickadeeapothecary.com/blogs/chickadee-apothecary/14660107-bramble-on-blackberry-wild-food-medicine>
7.   Chickadee Apothecary. "Bramble On, Blackberry: Wild Food & Medicine." June 14, 1016. Web. <https://www.chickadeeapothecary.com/blogs/chickadee-apothecary/14660107-bramble-on-blackberry-wild-food-medicine>
8.   Chickadee Apothecary. "Bramble On, Blackberry: Wild Food & Medicine." June 14, 2016. Web. <https://www.chickadeeapothecary.com/blogs/chickadee-apothecary/14660107-bramble-on-blackberry-wild-food-medicine>
9.   Jackson, Deb, and Karen Bergeron. Alternative Nature Online Herbal, "Blackberry Edible, Herbal use and Medicinal Properties." June 14, 2016. Web. <https://altnature.com/gallery/blackberry.htm>
10.   Chickadee Apothecary. "Bramble On, Blackberry: Wild Food & Medicine." June 14, 2016. Web. <https://www.chickadeeapothecary.com/blogs/chickadee-apothecary/14660107-bramble-on-blackberry-wild-food-medicine>
11.   Chickadee Apothecary. "Bramble On, Blackberry: Wild Food & Medicine." June 14, 2016. Web. <https://www.chickadeeapothecary.com/blogs/chickadee-apothecary/14660107-bramble-on-blackberry-wild-food-medicine>
12.   Chickadee Apothecary. "Bramble On, Blackberry: Wild Food & Medicine." June 14, 2016. Web. <https://www.chickadeeapothecary.com/blogs/chickadee-apothecary/14660107-bramble-on-blackberry-wild-food-medicine>
13.   Chickadee Apothecary. "Bramble On, Blackberry: Wild Food & Medicine." June 14, 2016. <https://www.chickadeeapothecary.com/blogs/chickadee-apothecary/14660107-bramble-on-blackberry-wild-food-medicine>
14.   "Rubus ameniacus." June 17, 2016. Web. <https://en.wikipedia.org/wiki/Rubus_armeniacus>
15.   Singing Nettles Herbal Clinic. "Early settlers used plants for food, medicine, and in the home." June 17, 2016. Web. <singingnettles.blogspot.com/2011/08/early-settlers-used-plants-for-food.html>
16.   Tryon Life Community Farm. "Blackberry (Rubus fruiticosus)-Native & Non-Native." June 14, 2016. Web. <tryonfarm.org/share/note/308>
17.   Jackson, Deb and Karen Bergeron. Alternative Nature Online Herbal. "Blackberry Edible, Herbal use and Medicinal Properties." June 14, 2016. Web. <https://altnature.com/gallery/blackberry.htm>
18.   Jackson, Deb and Karen Bergeron. Alternative Nature Online Herbal. "Blackberry Edible, Herbal use and Medicinal Properties." June 14, 2016. Web. <https://altnature.com/gallery/blackberry.htm>
19.   "Himalayan Blackberry." June 17, 2016. Web. <www.nwcb.wa.gov/site/Files/Rubus_armeniacus.pdf>

OTHER SOURCES:

Herbal Encyclopedia, "Blackberry." June 17, 2016. Web. <www.cloverleafarms.com/blackberry>

HORSETAIL

1. "Horsetail." August 7, 2015. Web. http://www.nlm.nih.gov/medlineplus/druginfo/natural843.htm>
2. "Horsetail: Herbal Remedies." August 7, 2015. Web. <health.howstuffworks.com/wellness/natural-medicine>
3. "Horsetail."August 7, 2017. Web. <http://www.nlm.nih.gov/medlineplus/druginfo/natural843.htm>
4. "Horsetail: Herbal Remedies." August 7, 2017. Web. <health.howstuffworks.com/wellness/natural-medicine>
5. "Horsetail: Herbal Remedies." August 7, 2017. Web. <health.howstuffworks.com/wellness/natural-medicine>
6. Homeremediesweb. "Horsetail Health Benefits." December 23, 2016. Web. <http://www.homeremediesweb.com/horsetail-health-benefits.php>
7. "Horsetail."August 7, 2015. Web. < http://www.nlm.nih.gov/medlineplus/druginfo/natural843.htm>
8. Homeremediesweb. "Horsetail Health Benefits." December 23, 2016. Web. <http://www.homeremediesweb.com/horsetail-health-benefits.php>
9. "Horsetail." August 7, 2015. Web. <http://www.nlm.nih.gov/medlineplus/druginfo/natural843.htm>
10. "Horsetail." August 7, 2015. Web. <http://www.nlm.nih.gov/medlineplus/druginfo/natural843.htm>
11. "Horsetail." August 7, 2015. Web. <http://www.nlm.nih.gov/medlineplus/druginfo/natural843.htm>
12. "Horsetail." August 7, 2015. Web. <http://www.nlm.nih.gov/medlineplus/druginfo/natural843.htm>
13. "Horsetail." August 7, 2015. Web. <http://www.nlm.nih.gov/medlineplus/druginfo/natural843.htm>
14. "Horsetail." August 7, 2015. Web. <http://www.nlm.nih.gov/medlineplus/druginfo/natural843.htm>
15. "Equisetum." August 7, 2015. Web. <https://en.wikipedia.org/wiki/Horsetail#spores>
16. Kelly, Erica and Richard Kissel. *Evolving Planet: Four Billion Years of Life on Earth.* Abrams Books for Young Readers. NY, NY: 2008.
17. John Laumer Design, Green Architecture. Treehugger. "Locally Grown Sandpaper: The Horsetail." August 24, 2006. Web. <http://www.treehugger.com/green-architecture/locally-grown-sandpaper-the-horsetail.html.>

OTHER SOURCES:
"Horsetail: Herbal Remedies." August 7, 2015. Web. <health.howstuffworks.com/wellness/natural-medicine>
"Equisetum." August 7, 2015. Web. <https://en.wikipedia.org/wiki/Horsetail#spores>

MALLOW

1. "Mallow (Malva parviflora) an Edible Friend." November 20, 2015. Web. <rootsimple.com/2008/02/mallow-malva-parviflora-an-edible-friend>
2. "Little Mallow (cheeseweed) (Malva parviflora)." November 20, 2015. Web. <ipm.com.ucdavis.edu/PMG/WEEDS/Little_Mallow.html>
3. "Medicinal herbs Cheeseweed Malva parviflora." November 20, 2015. Web. <naturalmedinalherbs.net/herbs/m/malva-parviflora=cheeseweed.php>
4. "Mallow (Malva parviflora) an Edible Friend." November 20, 2015. Web. <rootsimple.com/2008/02/mallow-malva-parviflora-an-edible-friend>
5. "Medicinal herbs Cheeseweed Malva parviflora." November 20, 2015. Web. <naturalmedinalherbs.net/herbs/m/malva-parviflora=cheeseweed.php>
6. "Medicinal herbs Cheeseweed Malva parviflora." November 20, 2015. Web. <naturalmedinalherbs.net/herbs/m/malva-parviflora=cheeseweed.php>
7. "Medicinal herbs Cheeseweed Malva parviflora." November 20, 2015. Web. <naturalmedinalherbs.net/herbs/m/malva-parviflora=cheeseweed.php>
8. Hall, Joan. Dengarden. "How to Find and Prepare Nutritious, Edible Mallows." November 22, 2015. Web. <https://dengarden.com/gardening/malva>
9. Hall, Joan. Dengarden, "How to Find and Prepare Nutritious, Edible Mallows." November 22, 2015. Web. <https://dengarden.com/gardening/malva>
10. "Weed Biology and Management." November 22, 2015. Web. <onlinelibrary.wiley.com/doi/101111/wbm.12063/abstract>
11. Hall, Joan. Dengarden, "How to Find and Prepare Nutritious, Edible Mallows." November 22, 2015. Web. <https://dengarden.com/gardening/malva>

12. "Nutritional Aspects of Wild Plants, Nutritional Composition of Malva parviflora and Sisybriumirio." November 22, 2015. Web. <agris.fao.org/agris-search.do?recordid=QC2004200201>
13. "Nutritional Aspects of Wild Plants, Nutritional Composition of Malva parviflora and Sisybriumirio." November 22, 2015. Web. <agris.fao.org/agris-search.do?recordid=QC2004200201>
14. Foraging Texas. "Mallow." November 22, 2015. Web. <foragingtexas.com/2008/08/Mallow.html>
15. "Malva parviflora Little Mallow." November 20, 2015. Web. <books.google.com/books>
16. "Weed Biology and Management." November 22, 2015. Web. <onlinelibrary.wiley.com/doi/101111/wbm.12063/abstract>

MILK THISTLE

1. WebMD. "Milk Thistle: Benefits and Side Effects." December 22, 2016. Web. <http://www.webmd.com/heart-disease/milk-thistle-benefits-and-side-effects#2>
2. Star Child. "Milk Thistle Seed *Silybum marianum*." December 22, 2016. Web. <http://www.starchild.co.uk/products/6564_3569_milk-thistle-seed-organic.aspx>
3. Dr. Axe. *Food Is Medicine*. "Milk Thistle Benefits: Detox the Liver & Boost Glutathione." January 1, 2017. Web. <draxe.com/milk-thistle-benefits>
4. WebMD. "Milk Thistle: Benefits and Side Effects." December 22, 2016. Web. <http://www.webmd.com/heart-disease/milk-thistle-benefits-and-side-effects#2>
5. Star Child. "Milk Thistle Seed *Silybum marianum*." December 22, 2016. Web. <http://www.starchild.co.uk/products/6564_3569_milk-thistle-seed-organic.aspx>
6. Star Child. "Milk Thistle Seed *Silybum marianum*." December 22, 2016. Web. <http://www.starchild.co.uk/products/6564_3569_milk-thistle-seed-organic.aspx>
7. Star Child. "Milk Thistle Seed *Silybum marianum*." December 22, 2016. Web. <http://www.starchild.co.uk/products/6564_3569_milk-thistle-seed-organic.aspx>
8. Star Child. "Milk Thistle Seed *Silybum marianum*." December 22, 2016. Web. <http://www.starchild.co.uk/products/6564_3569_milk-thistle-seed-organic.aspx>
9. Herbal Riot. "Magickal Uses of Milk Thistle." December 22, 2016. Web. <http://herbalriot.tumblr.com/post/67557549637/magickal-uses-of-milk-thistle>

MINER'S LETTUCE

1. The Atlantic. "Foraging for Miner's Lettuce, America's Gift to Salad." December 20, 2016. Web. <http://www.theatlantic.com/health/archive/2011/03/foraging-for-miners-lettuce-americas-gift-to-salad/72106>
2. The Atlantic. "Foraging for Miner's Lettuce, America's Gift to Salad." December 20, 2016. Web. <http://www.theatlantic.com/health/archive/2011/03/foraging-for-miners-lettuce-americas-gift-to-salad/72106>
3. Superfoods for Superhealth's Superfood Evolution. "Harvesting Miners Lettuce, a Wild Green Superfood." March 22, 2017. Web. <http://www.superfoods-for-superhealth.com/miners-lettuce.html>
4. Superfoods for Superhealth's Superfood Evolution, "Harvesting Miners Lettuce, a Wild Green Superfood." March 22, 2017. Web. <http://www.superfoods-for-superhealth.com/miners-lettuce.html>
5. "The Atlantic. "Foraging for Miner's Lettuce, America's Gift to Salad." December 20, 2016. Web. <http://www.theatlantic.com/health/archive/2011/03/foraging-for-miners-lettuce-americas-gift-to-salad/72106>
6. Superfoods for Superhealth's Superfood Evolution. "Harvesting Miners Lettuce, A Wild Green Superfood." March 22, 2017. Web. <http://www.superfoods-for-superhealth.com/miners-lettuce.html>
7. The Atlantic. "Foraging for Miner's Lettuce, America's Gift to Salad." December 20, 2016. Web. <http://www.theatlantic.com/health/archive/2011/03/foraging-for-miners-lettuce-americas-gift-to-salad/72106>
8. Superfoods for Superhealth's Superfood Evolution. "Harvesting Miners Lettuce, A Wild Green Superfood." March 17, 2017. Web. <http://www.superfoods-for-superhealth.com/miners-lettuce.html>
9. Herbs. "Miner's Lettuce." December 20, 2016. Web. <http://www.naturalmedicinalherbs.net/herbs/c/claytonia-perfoliata=miner's-lettuce.php>
10. Herbs. "Miner's Lettuce." December 20, 2016. Web. <http://www.naturalmedicinalherbs.net/herbs/c/claytonia-perfoliata=miner's-lettuce.php>
11. Wikipedia. "Claytonia perfoliata." December 20, 2016. Web. <https://en.wikipedia.org/wiki/Claytonia_perfoliata>
12. The Atlantic. "Foraging for Miner's Lettuce, America's Gift to Salad." December 20, 2016. Web. <http://www.theatlantic.com/health/archive/2011/03/foraging-for-miners-lettuce-americas-gift-to-salad/72106>

3. The Atlantic. "Foraging for Miner's Lettuce, America's Gift to Salad." December 20, 2016. Web. <http://www.theatlantic.com/health/archive/2011/03/foraging-for-miners-lettuce-americas-gift-to-salad/72106>

MUGWORT

1. The[Grow]network. "For the Love of Mugwort: 7 Uses for Mugwort." December 30, 2016. Web. <http://thegrownetwork.com/for-the-love-of-mugwort-7-uses-for-mugwort>
2. "Mugwort Herb-Uses and Side Effects" and "Native American Mugwort Mythology." August 10, 2015. Web. <best-home-remedies.com/herbal_medicine/herbs/mugwort.html>
3. The[Grow]network. "For the Love of Mugwort: 7 Uses for Mugwort." December 30, 2016. Web. <http://thegrownetwork.com/for-the-love-of-mugwort-7-uses-for-mugwort>
4. "Mugwort Herb-Uses and Side Effects" and "Native American Mugwort Mythology." August 10, 2015. Web. <best-home-remedies.com/herbal_medicine/herbs/mugwort.html>
5. The[Grow]network. "For the Love of Mugwort: 7 Uses for Mugwort." December 30, 2016. Web. <http://thegrownetwork.com/for-the-love-of-mugwort-7-uses-for-mugwort>
6. "Mugwort Herb-Uses and Side Effects" and "Native American Mugwort Mythology." August 10, 2015. Web. <best-home-remedies.com/herbal_medicine/herbs/mugwort.html>
7. The[Grow]network. "For the Love of Mugwort: 7 Uses for Mugwort." December 30, 2016. Web. <http://thegrownetwork.com/for-the-love-of-mugwort-7-uses-for-mugwort>
8. "Mugwort Herb-Uses and Side Effects" and "Native American Mugwort Mythology." August 10, 2015. Web. <best-home-remedies.com/herbal_medicine/herbs/mugwort.html>
9. "Mugwort Herb-Uses and Side Effects" and "Native American Mugwort Mythology." August 10, 2015. Web. <best-home-remedies.com/herbal_medicine/herbs/mugwort.html>
10. "Mugwort Herb-Uses and Side Effects" and "Native American Mugwort Mythology." August 10, 2015. Web. <best-home-remedies.com/herbal_medicine/herbs/mugwort.html>
11. Moore, Michael. *Medicinal Plants of the Pacific West.* Red Crane Books: Santa Fe, 1993.
12. Moore, Michael. *Medicinal Plants of the Pacific West.* Red Crane Books: Santa Fe, 1993.
13. The[Grow]network. "For the Love of Mugwort: 7 Uses for Mugwort." December 30, 2016. Web. <http://thegrownetwork.com/for-the-love-of-mugwort-7-uses-for-mugwort>
14. The[Grow]network. "For the Love of Mugwort: 7 Uses for Mugwort." December 30, 2016. Web. <http://thegrownetwork.com/for-the-love-of-mugwort-7-uses-for-mugwort>
15. Moore, Michael. *Medicinal Plants of the Pacific West.* Red Crane Books: Santa Fe, 1993.
16. The[Grow]network. "For the Love of Mugwort: 7 Uses for Mugwort." December 30, 2016. Web. <http://thegrownetwork.com/for-the-love-of-mugwort-7-uses-for-mugwort>
17. Moore, Michael. *Medicinal Plants of the Pacific West.* Red Crane Books: Santa Fe, 1993.
18. "Native American Mugwort Mythology." August 10, 2015. Web. <native-languages.org/legends-mugwort>
19. "Native American Mugwort Mythology." August 10, 2015. Web. <native-languages.org/legends-mugwort>
20. Acupucture Today. "Moxibustion." December 30, 2016. Web. <http://www.acupuncturetoday.com/abc/moxibustion.php>
21. Acupucture Today. "Moxibustion." December 30, 2016. Web. <http://www.acupuncturetoday.com/abc/moxibustion.php>
22. Acupucture Today, "Moxibustion." December 30, 2016. Web. <http://www.acupuncturetoday.com/abc/moxibustion.php>
23. Cupping Resource. "What is Moxibustion?" December 30, 2016. Web. <https://www.cuppingresource.com/what-is-moxibustion>
24. Serenaruns, "Using Traditional Chinese Medicine to Treat Warts." December 30, 2016. Web. <http://www.serenaruns.com/using-traditional-chinese-medicine-to-treat-warts>
25. Richters. "Praising the Artemisias!" December 30, 2016. Web. <https://www.richters.com/show.cgi?page=HerbOfTheYear/2014artemisia.html>

OTHER SOURCES:
Self-Heal School of Herbal Studies and Healing. "Mugwort-The Dream Herb." December 30, 2016. Web. <http://selfhealschool.com/mugwort>

PINEAPPLE WEED

1. Ethnobotany. "Pineapple Weed *Matricaria discoidea.*." March 11, 2017. Web. <http://winter2012bioportfolios.providence.wikispaces.net/Pineapple+weed>
2. Herbal Picnic. Guide to Herbal Remedies & Magic with Practical Recipes. "Pineapple Weed / Wild Chamomile." March 11, 2017. Web. <https://herbalpicnic.blogspot.com/2013/07/pineapple-weed-wild-chamomile.html>
3. "The Medicinal Properties of Chamomile (Pineapple Weed)" December 11, 2015. Web. <guidinginstincts.com/2012/06/medicinal-properties-of-chamomile.html>

4. Ethnobotany, "Pineapple Weed *Matricaria discoidea*." March 11, 2017. Web.
    <http://winter2012bioportfolios.providence.wikispaces.net/Pineapple+weed>
5. "The Medicinal Properties of Chamomile (Pineapple Weed)." December 11, 2015. Web.
    <guidinginstincts.com/2012/06/medicinal-properties-of-chamomile.html>
6. "The Medicinal Properties of Chamomile (Pineapple Weed)." December 11, 2015. Web.
    <guidinginstincts.com/2012/06/medicinal-properties-of-chamomile.html>
7. Ethnobotany, "Pineapple Weed *Matricaria discoidea*." March 11, 2017. Web.
    <http://winter2012bioportfolios.providence.wikispaces.net/Pineapple+weed>
8. "The Medicinal Properties of Chamomile (Pineapple Weed)." December 11, 2015. Web.
    <guidinginstincts.com/2012/06/medicinal-properties-of-chamomile.html>
9. "Midwest Permaculture." December 11, 2015. Web. <midwestpermaculture.com/2012/06/identifying-and-using-pineapple-weed-3>
10. "The Medicinal Properties of Chamomile (Pineapple Weed)." December 11, 2015
    <guidinginstincts.com/2012/06/medicinal-properties-of-chamomile.html>
11. "The Medicinal Properties of Chamomile (Pineapple Weed)." December 11, 2015. Web.
    <guidinginstincts.com/2012/06/medicinal-properties-of-chamomile.html>
12. Herbalpedia. "Pineapple Weed." December 19, 2015. Web.
    <http://www.herbworld.com/learningherbs/Pineapple%20Weed.pdf>
13. "The Medicinal Properties of Chamomile (Pineapple Weed)." December 11, 2015. Web.
    <guidinginstincts.com/2012/06/medicinal-properties-of-chamomile.html>
14. Herbal Picnic. Guide to Herbal Remedies & Magic with Practical Recipes. "Pineapple Weed / Wild
    Chamomile." March 11, 2017. Web. <https://herbalpicnic.blogspot.com/2013/07/pineapple-weed-wild-chamomile.html>
15. "Midwest Permaculture." December 11, 2015. Web. <midwestpermaculture.com/2012/06/identifying-and-using-pineapple-weed-3>
16. "Eat the Weeds and Other Things, Too, Pineapple Weed." March 11, 2017. Web.
    <eattheweeds.com/matricaria-matricarioides-for-your-tea-salad-2/comment-page-1>
17. "Midwest Permaculture." December 11, 2015. Web. <midwestpermaculture.com/2012/06/identifying-and-using-pineapple-weed-3>
18. Herbalpedia. "Pineapple Weed." December 19, 2015. Web.
    <http://www.herbworld.com/learningherbs/Pineapple%20Weed.pdf>
19. "Pineapple Weed." March 11, 2017. Web.
    <http://wildrootsherbs.homestead.com/pineapple_weed_09.pdf>
20. "Pineapple Weed." March 11, 2017. Web.
    <http://wildrootsherbs.homestead.com/pineapple_weed_09.pdf>
21. Nourishing Simplicity. "Herb Lesson #3 Pineapple Weed." March 20, 2017. Web.
    <http://nourishingsimplicity.org/2010/05/herb-lesson-3-pineapple-weed.html>
22. Herbalpedia. "Pineapple Weed." December 19, 2015. Web.
    <http://www.herbworld.com/learningherbs/Pineapple%20Weed.pdf>
23. "The Medicinal Properties of Chamomile (Pineapple Weed)." December 11, 2015. Web.
    <guidinginstincts.com/2012/06/medicinal-properties-of-chamomile.html>
24. "The Medicinal Properties of Chamomile (Pineapple Weed) ." December 11, 2015. Web.
    <guidinginstincts.com/2012/06/medicinal-properties-of-chamomile.html>
25. "The Medicinal Properties of Chamomile (Pineapple Weed) ." December 11, 2015. Web.
    <guidinginstincts.com/2012/06/medicinal-properties-of-chamomile.html>
26. Herbalpedia. "Pineapple Weed." December 19, 2015. Web.
    <http://www.herbworld.com/learningherbs/Pineapple%20Weed.pdf>
27. Herbalpedia. "Pineapple Weed." December 19, 2015. Web.
    <http://www.herbworld.com/learningherbs/Pineapple%20Weed.pdf>
28. "Midwest Permaculture." December 11, 2015. Web. <midwestpermaculture.com/2012/06/identifying-and-using-pineapple-weed-3>
29. "Midwest Permaculture." December 11, 2015. Web. <midwestpermaculture.com/2012/06/identifying-and-using-pineapple-weed-3>

OTHER SOURCES:
"Plants For A Future." December 11, 2015. Web. <pfaf.org/user/Plant.aspx? LatinName-Matricaria+matricarioides>
"Eat the Weeds and other things, too, Pineapple Weed." March 11, 2017. Web. <eattheweeds.com/matricaria-matricarioides-for-your-tea-salad-2/comment-page-1>
NatureGate. "Pineapple Mayweed
Matricaria discoidea." March 11, 2017. Web. <http://www.luontoportti.com/suomi/en/kukkakasvit/pineapple-mayweed>

. Belebuono, Holly. *The Essential Herbal for Natural Health: How to Transform Easy-to-Find Herbs into Healing Remedies for the Whole Family.* Boston Ma: Roost Books, 2012.

. Wellness Mama. Simple Answers for Healthier Families, "Plantain: A Healing Herb in Your Backyard." December 31, 2016 . Web. < https://wellnessmama.com/5387/plantain-healing-herb>

. Skenderi, Gazmund. "Plantain." *Herbal Vade Mecum.* Rutherford, New Jersey; Herbacy Press, 2003. Page 300.

. Tierra, Lesley. *Healing With the Herbs of Life.* Berkley, CA: Ten Speed Press, 2003.

. Wellness Mama. Simple Answers for Healthier Families. "Plantain: A Healing Herb in Your Backyard." December 31, 2016 . Web. < https://wellnessmama.com/5387/plantain-healing-herb>

. Skenderi, Gazmund. "Plantain." *Herbal Vade Mecum.* Rutherford, New Jersey; Herbacy Press, 2003. Page 300.

. Belebuono, Holly. *The Essential Herbal for Natural health: How to Transform Easy-to-Find herbs into Healing Remedies for the Whole Family.* Boston Ma: Roost Books, 2012.

. Skenderi, Gazmund. "Plantain." *Herbal Vade Mecum.* Rutherford, New Jersey; Herbacy Press, 2003. Page 300.

. Skenderi, Gazmund. "Plantain." *Herbal Vade Mecum.* Rutherford, New Jersey; Herbacy Press, 2003. Page 300.

10. Moore, Michael. "Plantain." *Medicinal Plants of the Pacific West.* Santa Fe, NM: Red Crane Books, 1993. Page 303.

11. Indian Journal of Traditional Knowledge. "A Review of the Plantago Plant." Vol. 13 (4), October, 2014. December 31, 2016. Web. pp. 681-685. <http://nopr.niscair.res.in/bitstream/123456789/29518/1/IJTK%2013(4)%20681-685.pdf>

12. Skenderi, Gazmund. *Herbal Vade Mecum.* "Plantain." Herbacy Press, Rutherford, New Jersey; 2003. Page 300.

13. Indian Journal of Traditional Knowledge. "A Review of the Plantago Plant." Vol. 13 (4), October, 2014. December 31, 2016. Web. pp. 681-685. <http://nopr.niscair.res.in/bitstream/123456789/29518/1/IJTK%2013(4)%20681-685.pdf>

14. Skenderi, Gazmund. *Herbal Vade Mecum.* "Plantain." Herbacy Press, Rutherford, New Jersey; 2003. Page 300.

15. Belebuono, Holly. *The Essential Herbal for Natural Health: How to Transform Easy-to-Find Herbs into Healing Remedies for the Whole Family.* Boston Ma: Roost Books, 2012.

16. Skenderi, Gazmund. *Herbal Vade Mecum.* "Plantain." Herbacy Press, Rutherford, New Jersey; 2003. Page 300.

17. Prota4U. "Plantago lanceolata L." December 31, 2016. Web. <http://www.prota4u.org/protav8.asp?en=1&p=Plantago+lanceolata+L.>

18. Prota4U. "Plantago lanceolata L." December 31, 2016. Web. <http://www.prota4u.org/protav8.asp?en=1&p=Plantago+lanceolata+L.>

19. Ahlborn, Margaret L. *Dr. Christopher's Herbal Legacy,* "History of Plantain." < http://www.herballegacy.com/Ahlborn_History.html> December 31, 2016

20. Wellness Mama. Simple Answers for Healthier Families. "Plantain: A Healing Herb in Your Backyard." December 31, 2016 . Web. < https://wellnessmama.com/5387/plantain-healing-herb>

21. Ahlborn, Margeret L. *Dr. Christopher's Herbal Legacy.* December 31, 2016. Web. "History of Plantain." <http://www.herballegacy.com/Ahlborn_History.html>

22. Ahlborn, Margeret L. *Dr. Christopher's Herbal Legacy.* December 31, 2016. Web. "History of Plantain." <http://www.herballegacy.com/Ahlborn_History.html>

23. Wellness Mama. Simple Answers for Healthier Families. "Plantain: A Healing Herb in Your Backyard." December 31, 2016 . Web. < https://wellnessmama.com/5387/plantain-healing-herb>

24. Ahlborn, Margeret L. *Dr. Christopher's Herbal Legacy.* December 31, 2016. Web. "History of Plantain." <http://www.herballegacy.com/Ahlborn_History.html>

25. Ahlborn, Margeret L. *Dr. Christopher's Herbal Legacy.* December 31, 2016. Web. "History of Plantain." <http://www.herballegacy.com/Ahlborn_History.html>

REDWOOD

1. Moore, Michael. "Redwood." *Medicinal Plants of the Pacific West.* Santa Fe, NM: Red Crane Books, 1993. 219-221.

2. Bay Nature: An Exploration of Nature in the San Francisco Bay Area. "Fog and redwoods: Demystifying the Mist." December 20, 2016. Web. <baynature.org/article/fog-and-redwoods-demystifying-the-mist>

3. Moore, Michael. "Redwood." *Medicinal Plants of the Pacific West*. Santa Fe, NM: Red Crane Books, 1993.

4. Spirit Weavers Gathering. "Medicine of the Forest: The Great Redwood Beings." December 26, 2016. Web. <http://www.spiritweaversgathering.com/medicine-of-the-forest-the-great-redwood-beings>

5. Moore, Michael. "Redwood." *Medicinal Plants of the Pacific West*. Santa Fe, NM: Red Crane Books, 1993. 219-221.

6. Grow Forage Cook Ferment. "Foraging for Pine Needles (and Other Conifer Needles)." December 21, 2016. Web. <www.growforagecookferment.com/foraging-for-pine-needles>

7. Spirit Weavers Gathering. "Medicine of the Forest: The Great Redwood Beings." December 26, 2016. Web. <http://www.spiritweaversgathering.com/medicine-of-the-forest-the-great-redwood-beings>

8. Moore, Michael. "Redwood." *Medicinal Plants of the Pacific West*. Santa Fe, NM: Red Crane Books, 1993. 219-221.

9. Grow Forage Cook Ferment. "Foraging for Pine Needles (and Other Conifer Needles)." December 21, 2016. Web. <www.growforagecookferment.com/foraging-for-pine-needles>

10. Spirit Weavers Gathering. "Medicine of the Forest: The Great Redwood Beings." December 26, 2016. Web. <http://www.spiritweaversgathering.com/medicine-of-the-forest-the-great-redwood-beings>

11. Grow Forage Cook Ferment. "Foraging for Pine Needles (and Other Conifer Needles)." December 21, 2016. Web. <www.growforagecookferment.com/foraging-for-pine-needles>

12. Illustrated Native Ethnobotany of Coastal Northern California, <http://www.asis.com/users/jknope/redwood.html> December 21, 2016

13. Spirit Weavers Gathering. "Medicine of the Forest: The Great Redwood Beings." December 26, 2016. Web. <http://www.spiritweaversgathering.com/medicine-of-the-forest-the-great-redwood-beings>

14. National Park Service. "Redwood." December 21, 2015. Web. <http://www.nps.gov/redw/learn/history culture/area-history.htm>

15. National Park Service. "Redwood." December 21, 2015. Web. <http://www.nps.gov/redw/learn/history culture/area-history.htm>

16. National Park Service. "Redwood." December 21, 2015. Web. <http://www.nps.gov/redw/learn/history culture/area-history.htm>

17. First Peoples. "California Big Trees: A Paiute Legend." December 21, 2015. Web. <http://www.firstpeople.us/FP-Html-Legends/CaliforniaBigTrees.Paiute.html>

18. Los Padres Forest Watch. "Coast Redwood, Sequoia Sempervirens." December 27, 2015. Web. <http://www.lpfw.org/archive/about/critters/coastredwood.htm>

SOUR GRASS

1. Wikipedia. "Oxalidaceae." March 19, 2017. Web. <https://en.wikipedia.org/wiki/Oxalidaceae>

2. Murrey, HMHarrison. "Wild Edibles-The Delicious, Lemony, Medicinal Wood Sorrel." March 19, 2017. Web. <http://bushcraftskills.blogspot.com/2010/07/wild-edibles-delicious-lemony-medicinal.html>

3. Elpel, Thomas. *Botany in a Day*. Hops Press: Toby, MT, 2013.

4. Mercury News. "Master Gardener: Get a Jump on Oxalis." March 19, 2017. Web. <http://www.mercurynews.com/2010/12/06/master-gardener-get-a-jump-on-oxalis>

5. Murrey, HMHarrison. "Wild Edibles-The Delicious, Lemony, Medicinal Wood Sorrel." March 19, 2017. Web. <http://bushcraftskills.blogspot.com/2010/07/wild-edibles-delicious-lemony-medicinal.html>

6. Murrey, HMHarrison. "Wild Edibles-The Delicious, Lemony, Medicinal Wood Sorrel." March 19, 2017. Web. <http://bushcraftskills.blogspot.com/2010/07/wild-edibles-delicious-lemony-medicinal.html>

7. Gardens ablaze. "Medicinal Uses of Oxalis (Wood Sorrel)." March 19, 2017. Web. <http://www.gardensablaze.com/HerbOxalisMed.htm>

8. Murrey, HMHarrison. "Wild Edibles-The Delicious, Lemony, Medicinal Wood Sorrel." March 19, 2017. Web. <http://bushcraftskills.blogspot.com/2010/07/wild-edibles-delicious-lemony-medicinal.html>

9. Alternative Nature Online Herbal. "Wood Sorrel Herb." March 19, 2017. Web. <https://altnature.com/gallery/woodsorrel.htm>

10. Alternative Nature Online Herbal, "Wood Sorrel Herb." March 19, 2017. Web. <https://altnature.com/gallery/woodsorrel.htm>

11. Murrey, HMHarrison. "Wild Edibles-The Delicious, Lemony, Medicinal Wood Sorrel." March 19, 2017. Web. <http://bushcraftskills.blogspot.com/2010/07/wild-edibles-delicious-lemony-medicinal.html>

12. Alternative Nature Online Herbal, "Wood Sorrel Herb." March 19, 2017. Web. <https://altnature.com/gallery/woodsorrel.htm>

13. Murrey, HMHarrison. "Wild Edibles-The Delicious, Lemony, Medicinal Wood Sorrel." March 19, 2017. Web. <http://bushcraftskills.blogspot.com/2010/07/wild-edibles-delicious-lemony-medicinal.html>

14. Alternative Nature Online Herbal, "Wood Sorrel Herb." March 19, 2017. Web. <https://altnature.com/gallery/woodsorrel.htm>

5. Gardens ablaze, "Medicinal Uses of Oxalis (Wood Sorrel)." March 19, 2017. Web. <http://www.gardensablaze.com/HerbOxalisMed.htm>
6. Gardens ablaze, "Medicinal Uses of Oxalis (Wood Sorrel)." March 19, 2017. Web. <http://www.gardensablaze.com/HerbOxalisMed.htm>
7. One Writer's Way. "Herbal Lore: Wood Sorrel, Oxalis, and the Shamrock–Beth Trissel." March 19, 2017. Web. <bethtrissel.wordpress.com/2013/03/17/herbal-lore-wood-sorrel-oxalis-and-the-shamrock-beth-trissel>
8. Alternative Nature Online Herbal. "Wood Sorrel Herb." March 19, 2017. Web. <https://altnature.com/gallery/woodsorrel.htm>
9. Alternative Nature Online Herbal, "Wood Sorrel Herb." March 19, 2017. Web. <https://altnature.com/gallery/woodsorrel.htm>
20. Alternative Nature Online Herbal, "Wood Sorrel Herb." March 19, 2017. Web. <https://altnature.com/gallery/woodsorrel.htm>
21. Wikipedia. "Potassium hydrogenoxalate." March 19, 2017. Web. <https://en.wikipedia.org/wiki/Potassium_hydrogenoxalate>
22. Gardens Ablaze. "Medicinal Uses of Oxalis (Wood Sorrel)." March 19, 2017. Web. <http://www.gardensablaze.com/HerbOxalisMed.htm>
23. Murrey, HMHarrison. "Wild Edibles-The Delicious, Lemony, Medicinal Wood Sorrel." March 19, 2017. Web. <http://bushcraftskills.blogspot.com/2010/07/wild-edibles-delicious-lemony-medicinal.html>
24. Healthy Wild & Free. "This is Why You Should Cook Your Spinach Before You Eat It." March 19, 2017. Web. <https://healthywildandfree.com/this-is-why-you-should-cook-your-spinach-before-you-eat-it/>
25. Healthy Wild & Free. "This is Why You Should Cook Your Spinach Before You Eat It." March 19, 2017. Web. <https://healthywildandfree.com/this-is-why-you-should-cook-your-spinach-before-you-eat-it/>
26. Murrey, HMHarrison. "Wild Edibles-The Delicious, Lemony, Medicinal Wood Sorrel." March 19, 2017. Web. <http://bushcraftskills.blogspot.com/2010/07/wild-edibles-delicious-lemony-medicinal.html>
27. Murrey, HMHarrison. "Wild Edibles-The Delicious, Lemony, Medicinal Wood Sorrel." March 19, 2017. Web. <http://bushcraftskills.blogspot.com/2010/07/wild-edibles-delicious-lemony-medicinal.html>
28. Gardens Ablaze. "Medicinal Uses of Oxalis (Wood Sorrel)." <http://www.gardensablaze.com/HerbOxalisMed.htm>
29. Mercury News. "Master Gardener: Get a Jump on Oxalis." March 19, 2017. Web. <http://www.mercurynews.com/2010/12/06/master-gardener-get-a-jump-on-oxalis>
30. Wikipedia. "Shamrock." March 19, 2017. Web. <https://en.wikipedia.org/wiki/Shamrock>
31. One Writer's Way. "Herbal Lore: Wood Sorrel, Oxalis, and the Shamrock–Beth Trissel." March 19, 2017. Web. <bethtrissel.wordpress.com/2013/03/17/herbal-lore-wood-sorrel-oxalis-and-the-shamrock-beth-trissel>
32. One Writer's Way. "Herbal Lore: Wood Sorrel, Oxalis, and the Shamrock–Beth Trissel." March 19, 2017. Web. <bethtrissel.wordpress.com/2013/03/17/herbal-lore-wood-sorrel-oxalis-and-the-shamrock-beth-trissel>
33. Murrey, HMHarrison. "Wild Edibles-The Delicious, Lemony, Medicinal Wood Sorrel." March 19, 2017. Web. <http://bushcraftskills.blogspot.com/2010/07/wild-edibles-delicious-lemony-medicinal.html>
34. Murrey, HMHarrison. "Wild Edibles-The Delicious, Lemony, Medicinal Wood Sorrel." March 19, 2017. Web. <http://bushcraftskills.blogspot.com/2010/07/wild-edibles-delicious-lemony-medicinal.html>
35. Alternative Nature Online Herbal. "Wood Sorrel Herb." March 19, 2017. Web. <https://altnature.com/gallery/woodsorrel.htm>
36. Murrey, HMHarrison. "Wild Edibles-The Delicious, Lemony, Medicinal Wood Sorrel." March 19, 2017. Web. <http://bushcraftskills.blogspot.com/2010/07/wild-edibles-delicious-lemony-medicinal.html>
37. Alternative Nature Online Herbal. "Wood Sorrel Herb." March 19, 2017. Web. <https://altnature.com/gallery/woodsorrel.htm>
38. University of Nebraska-Lincoln. "Yellow Woodsorrel." July 3, 2017. Web. <http://communityenvironment.unl.edu/yellow-woodsorrel>

ST. JOHN'S WORT

1. Moore, Michael. "Hypericum." *Medicinal Plants of the Pacific West*. Santa Fe, NM: Red Crane Books, 1993. Pages 153-156.

2. NCBI. "Chapter 11, Medical Attributes of St. John's Wort (*Hypericum perforatum*)." *Herbal Medicine: Biomolecular and Clinical Aspects. 2nd edition.* Dec. 24, 2016. Web. <ncbi.nlm.nih.gov/books/NBK92750>

3. Moore, Michael. "Hypericum." *Medicinal Plants of the Pacific West.* Santa Fe, NM: Red Crane Books, 1993. Page 153-156.

4. Moore, Michael. "Hypericum." *Medicinal Plants of the Pacific West.* Santa Fe, NM: Red Crane Books, 1993. Pages 153-156.

5. Moore, Michael. "Hypericum." *Medicinal Plants of the Pacific West.* Santa Fe, NM: Red Crane Books, 1993. Pages 153-156.

6. NCBI. "Chapter 11, Medical Attributes of St. John's Wort (*Hypericum perforatum*)." *Herbal Medicine: Biomolecular and Clinical Aspects. 2nd edition.* December 24, 2016. Web. <https://www.ncbi.nlm.nih.gov/books/NBK92750>

7. Moore, Michael. "Hypericum." *Medicinal Plants of the Pacific West.* Santa Fe, NM: Red Crane Books, 1993. Pages 153-156.

8. WebMD, "St. John's Wort." < http://www.webmd.com/vitamins-supplements/ingredientmono-329st%20john%27s%20wort.aspx?activeingredientid=329&activeingredientname=st%20john%27s%20wort> March 20, 2017

9. Moore, Michael. "Hypericum." *Medicinal Plants of the Pacific West.* Santa Fe, NM: Red Crane Books, 1993. Pages 153-156.

10. Moore, Michael. "Hypericum." *Medicinal Plants of the Pacific West.* Santa Fe, NM: Red Crane Books, 1993. Pages 153-156.

11. Moore, Michael. "Hypericum." *Medicinal Plants of the Pacific West.* Santa Fe, NM: Red Crane Books, 1993. Pages 153-156.

12. WebMD. "St. John's Wort." March 20, 2017. Web. < http://www.webmd.com/vitamins-supplements/ingredientmono-329st%20john%27s%20wort.aspx?activeingredientid=329&activeingredientname=st%20john%27s%20wort>

13. NCBI. "Chapter 11, Medical Attributes of St. John's Wort (*Hypericum perforatum*)." *Herbal Medicine: Biomolecular and Clinical Aspects. 2nd edition.* December 24, 2016. Web. <https://www.ncbi.nlm.nih.gov/books/NBK92750>

14. NCBI. "Chapter 11, Medical Attributes of St. John's Wort (*Hypericum perforatum*)." *Herbal Medicine: Biomolecular and Clinical Aspects. 2nd edition.* December 24, 2016. Web. <https://www.ncbi.nlm.nih.gov/books/NBK92750>

15. Hobbs, Christopher Ph.D., L.Ac., A.H.G. "St. John's Wort: A Review." December 24, 2016. Web. <http://www.christopherhobbs.com/library/articles-on-herbs-and-health/st-johns-wort-a-review>

STINGING NETTLE

1. DailyMail. "Why DO Stinging Nettles Hurt So Much? Chemist Shows How Tiny Hairs Inject Venom to Produce Pain - and Dock Leaves DON'T Help." December 28, 2016. Web. <http://www.dailymail.co.uk/sciencetech/article-3112201/Why-stinging-nettles-hurt-Chemist-shows-tiny-hairs-inject-venom-produce-pain-dock-leaves-WON-T-help.html>

2. The Radicle Review. "Notes from the Undergrowth: 'Nettles for Bleeding.'" December 28, 2016. Web. <https://theradiclereview.com/tag/nettles-for-bleeding>

3. The Radicle Review. "Notes from the Undergrowth: 'Nettles for Bleeding.'" December 28, 2016. Web. <https://theradiclereview.com/tag/nettles-for-bleeding>

4. University of Maryland Medical Center. "Stinging Nettle." July 24, 2015. Web. <umm.edu/health/medical/altmed/herb/Stinging-Nettle>

5. The Radicle Review. "Notes from the Undergrowth: 'Nettles for Bleeding.'" December 28, 2016. Web. <https://theradiclereview.com/tag/nettles-for-bleeding>

6. University of Maryland Medical Center. "Stinging Nettle." July 24, 2015. Web. <umm.edu/health/medical/altmed/herb/Stinging-Nettle>

7. Moore, Michael. "Nettle." *Medicinal Plants of the Pacific West.* Red Crane Books: Santa Fe, 1993. Pages 185 – 190.

8. The Radicle Review. "Notes from the Undergrowth: 'Nettles for Bleeding.'" December 28, 2016. Web. < https://theradiclereview.com/tag/nettles-for-bleeding>

9. Moore, Michael. "Nettle." *Medicinal Plants of the Pacific West.* Red Crane Books: Santa Fe, 1993. Pages 185 – 190.

10. Moore, Michael. "Nettle." *Medicinal Plants of the Pacific West.* Red Crane Books: Santa Fe, 1993. Pages 185 – 190.

11. Moore, Michael. "Nettle." *Medicinal Plants of the Pacific West.* Red Crane Books: Santa Fe, 1993. Pages 185 – 190.

2. University of Maryland Medical Center. "Stinging Nettle." July 24, 2015. Web. <umm.edu/health/medical/altmed/herb/Stinging-Nettle>
3. Moore, Michael. "Nettle." *Medicinal Plants of the Pacific West*. Red Crane Books: Santa Fe, 1993. Pages 185 – 190.
4. Vance, Kassie. "Stinging Nettle." July 25, 2015. Web. <herballegacy.com/Vance_StingingNettle.html>
5. Vance, Kassie. "Stinging Nettle." July 25, 2015. Web. <herballegacy.com/Vance_StingingNettle.html>

WILD OATS

1. "Avena fatua L. Poceae (Grass Family) Europe Wild Oat." February 24, 2017. Web. <http://nathistoc.bio.uci.edu/Plants%20of%20Upper%20Newport%20Bay%20(Robert%20De%20Ruff)/Poaceae/Avena%20fatua.htm>
2. MDidea. "Health Benefits, Effects and Pharmacological Findings of Oat Straw." February 24, 2017. Web. <https://www.mdidea.com/products/new/new03207.html>
3. MDidea. "Health Benefits, Effects and Pharmacological Findings of Oat Straw." February 24, 2017. Web. <https://www.mdidea.com/products/new/new03207.html>
4. "Wild Edible and Medicinal Plants: Using What Nature Provides in Plants." February 24, 2017. Web. <https://keys2liberty.wordpress.com/tag/avena-fatua>
5. "Wild Edible and Medicinal Plants: Using What Nature Provides in Plants." February 24, 2017. Web. <https://keys2liberty.wordpress.com/tag/avena-fatua>
6. Herbwisdom. "Avena Sativa-Oats." September 28, 2015. Web. <http://www.herbwisdom.com/herb-avena-sativa.html>
7. MDidea. "Health Benefits, Effects and Pharmacological Findings of Oat Straw." February 24, 2017. Web. <https://www.mdidea.com/products/new/new03207.html>
8. California School of Herbal Studies. "Wild Oats, Common Oats, Catgrass." September 27, 2015. Web. <http://www.cshs.com/herbsOfMonth/oats.html>
9. MDidea. "Health Benefits, Effects and Pharmacological Findings of Oat Straw." February 24, 2017. Web. <https://www.mdidea.com/products/new/new03207.html>
10. MDidea. "Health Benefits, Effects and Pharmacological Findings of Oat Straw." February 24, 2017. Web. <https://www.mdidea.com/products/new/new03207.html>
11. California School of Herbal Studies. "Wild Oats, Common Oats, Catgrass." September 27, 2015. Web. <http://www.cshs.com/herbsOfMonth/oats.html>
12. "Avena fatua L. Poceae (Grass Family) Europe Wild Oat." February 24, 2017. Web. <http://nathistoc.bio.uci.edu/Plants%20of%20Upper%20Newport%20Bay%20(Robert%20De%20Ruff)/Poaceae/Avena%20fatua.htm>
13. California School of Herbal Studies. "Wild Oats, Common Oats, Catgrass." September 27, 2015. Web. <http://www.cshs.com/herbsOfMonth/oats.html>
14. California's Coastal Prairies. "Early Europeans, Ranches, Agriculture, Invasive Plants." September 27, 2015. Web. <http://sonoma.edu/cei/prairie/history/recent_history.html>
15. California's Coastal Prairies. "Early Europeans, Ranches, Agriculture, Invasive Plants." September 27, 2015. Web. <http://sonoma.edu/cei/prairie/history/recent_history.html>
16. California's Coastal Prairies. "Early Europeans, Ranches, Agriculture, Invasive Plants." September 27, 2015. Web. <http://sonoma.edu/cei/prairie/history/recent_history.html>
17. California's Coastal Prairies. "Early Europeans, Ranches, Agriculture, Invasive Plants." September 27, 2015. Web. <http://sonoma.edu/cei/prairie/history/recent_history.html>
18. California's Coastal Prairies. "Early Europeans, Ranches, Agriculture, Invasive Plants." September 27, 2015. Web. <http://sonoma.edu/cei/prairie/history/recent_history.html>
19. "Avena fatua L. Poceae (Grass Family) Europe Wild Oat." February 24, 2017. Web. <http://nathistoc.bio.uci.edu/Plants%20of%20Upper%20Newport%20Bay%20(Robert%20De%20Ruff)/Poaceae/Avena%20fatua.htm>
20. Wikipedia. "Cahuila." February 24, 2017. Web. <https://en.wikipedia.org/wiki/Cahuilla>
21. "Avena fatua L. Poceae (Grass Family) Europe Wild Oat." February 24, 2017. Web. <http://nathistoc.bio.uci.edu/Plants%20of%20Upper%20Newport%20Bay%20(Robert%20De%20Ruff)/Poaceae/Avena%20fatua.htm>
22. Wikipedia. "Cahuila." February 24, 2017. Web. <https://en.wikipedia.org/wiki/Cahuilla>
23. California School of Herbal Studies. "Wild Oats, Common Oats, Catgrass." September 27, 2015. Web. <http://www.cshs.com/herbsOfMonth/oats.html>

OTHER SOURCES:
Michigan Medicine University of Michigan. "Oats." February 24, 2017. Web. <http://www.uofmhealth.org/health-library/hn-2138000>

US National Library of Medicine National Institutes of Health. "Chronic Effects of a Wild Green Oat Extract Supplementation on Cognitive Performance in Older Adults: A Randomised, Double-Blind, Placebo-Controlled, Crossover Trial." February 24, 2017. Web.
< https://www.ncbi.nlm.nih.gov/pmc/articles/PMC3367260>
Plants For A Future. "Avena fatua-L." February 24, 2017. Web.
<http://pfaf.org/user/Plant.aspx?LatinName=Avena+fatua>
The Woman's Roots. "Sweet Cream: The Medicine of Milky Oats." February 24, 2017. Web.
<http://bearmedicineherbals.com/sweet-cream-the-medicine-of-milky-oats.html>
The Dr. Oz Show. "Oat Straw Fact Sheet." February 24, 2017. Web. <http://www.doctoroz.com/article/oat-straw-fact-sheet>

WILLOW

1. Wild Foods & Medicines. "Willow." December 23, 2016. Web.
<http://wildfoodsandmedicines.com/willow>
2. University of Maryland Medical Center. "Willow Bark." February 16, 2016. Web.
<umm.edu/health/medical/altmed/herb/willow-bark>
3. Home Remedies. "Willow." March 13, 2016. Web. < http://home-remedies.com/willow>
4. University of Maryland Medical Center. "Willow Bark." February 16, 2016. Web.
<umm.edu/health/medical/altmed/herb/willow-bark>
5. University of Maryland Medical Center. "Willow Bark." February 16, 2016. Web.
<umm.edu/health/medical/altmed/herb/willow-bark>
6. Medical Herbs Info. "Willow." December 23, 2016. Web.
<http://medicinalherbinfo.org/herbs/Willow.html>
7. Medical Herbs Info. "Willow." December 23, 2016. Web.
<http://medicinalherbinfo.org/herbs/Willow.html>
8. University of Maryland Medical Center. "Willow Bark." February 16, 2016. Web.
<umm.edu/health/medical/altmed/herb/willow-bark>
9. Skenderi, Gazmund. *Herbal Vade Mecum*. Rutherford, New Jersey; Herbacy Press, 2003.
10. Wild Foods & Medicines. "Willow." December 23, 2016. Web.
<http://wildfoodsandmedicines.com/willow>
11. "White Willow, *Salix Alba*." February 17, 2016. Web. <anniesremedy.com/herb_detail62php>
12. Trees For Life. "Willow." March 13, 2016. Web. <Treesforlife.org.uk/forest/mythology-folklore/willow>
13. Trees For Life. "Willow." March 13, 2016. Web. <Treesforlife.org.uk/forest/mythology-folklore/willow>
14. Trees For Life. "Willow." March 13, 2016. Web. <Treesforlife.org.uk/forest/mythology-folklore/willow>
15. Trees For Life. "Willow." March 13, 2016. Web. <Treesforlife.org.uk/forest/mythology-folklore/willow>
16. Prindle, Tara. "Native American Technology and Art: Willow Branches and Other Twigs and Roots."
March 21, 2017. Web. <http://www.nativetech.org/willow/willow.htm>
17. Wild Foods & Medicines. "Willow." December 23, 2016. Web.
<http://wildfoodsandmedicines.com/willow>

OTHER SOURCES:
Plants of Southern California, "Salix: Key to Willows of Coastal Southern California Below 6000 Feet Elevation
<tchester.org/plants/analysis/salix/key.html> February 16, 2016
"White Willow Salix Alba." <anniesremedy.com/herb_detail62php> February 17, 2016
"Historical review of Medicinal Plant's Usage." <ncbi.nlm.nih.gov/pmc/articles/prk33558962> March 5, 2016

YARROW

1. Gladstar, Rosemary. "Yarrow *Achillea millefolium* Compositae Parts Used: Leaves and Flowers." *Herbal Healing for Women: Simple Home Remedies for Women of All Ages*. New York, NY: Fireside, 1993. Pages 259-260.
2. Falconi, Dina. *Earthly Bodies and Heavenly Hair: Natural and Healthy Personal Care for Every Body*. Ceres Press: Woodstock, New York, 1998.
3. Moore, Michael. "Yarrow." *Medicinal Plants of the Pacific West*. Santa Fe, NM: Red Crane Books, 1993. Pages 272-275.
4. Falconi, Dina. *Earthly Bodies and Heavenly Hair: Natural and Healthy Personal Care for Every Body*. Ceres Press: Woodstock, New York, 1998.
5. Herbs2000. "Yarrow Achillea millefolium." January 29, 2017. Web.
<http://www.herbs2000.com/herbs/herbs_yarrow.htm>
6. Sacred Earth Ethnobotany and Ecotravel. "Yarrow Achillea millefolium Compositae." January 29, 2017. Web. <http://www.sacredearth.com/ethnobotany/plantprofiles/yarrow.php>
7. Herbs2000. "Yarrow Achillea millefolium." January 29, 2017. Web.
<http://www.herbs2000.com/herbs/herbs_yarrow.htm>
8. Homemade Medicine. "Home Remedies Bleeding." January 29, 2017. Web.
<https://www.homemademedicine.com/home-remedies-bleeding.html>
9. Moore, Michael. "Yarrow." *Medicinal Plants of the Pacific West*. Santa Fe, NM: Red Crane Books, 1993. Pages 272-275.
10. Homemade Medicine. "Home Remedies Bleeding." January 29, 2017. Web.
<https://www.homemademedicine.com/home-remedies-bleeding.html>

1. Herbs2000. "Yarrow Achillea millefolium." January 29, 2017. Web. <http://www.herbs2000.com/herbs/herbs_yarrow.htm>
2. Herbs2000. "Yarrow Achillea millefolium." January 29, 2017. Web. <http://www.herbs2000.com/herbs/herbs_yarrow.htm>
3. Herbs2000. "Yarrow Achillea millefolium." January 29, 2017. Web. <http://www.herbs2000.com/herbs/herbs_yarrow.htm>
4. Herbs2000. "Yarrow Achillea millefolium." January 29, 2017. Web. <http://www.herbs2000.com/herbs/herbs_yarrow.htm>
5. Weed, Susun S. "Childbearing & Mothering ... Bladder Infections." *Wise Woman Herbal Ezine with Susan Weed.* January 29, 2017. Web. <http://www.susunweed.com/herbal_ezine/February08/childbearing.htm>
16. Herbs2000. "Yarrow Achillea millefolium." January 29, 2017. Web. <http://www.herbs2000.com/herbs/herbs_yarrow.htm>
17. Herbs2000. "Yarrow Achillea millefolium." January 29, 2017. Web. <http://www.herbs2000.com/herbs/herbs_yarrow.htm>
18. Sunnyfield Herb Farm Indispensible Herbs. "Achillea millefolium. Yarrow." January 29, 2017. Web. <http://www.matthewwoodherbs.com/Yarrow.html>
19. Sunnyfield Herb Farm Indispensible Herbs, "Achillea millefolium. Yarrow." January 29, 2017. Web. <http://www.matthewwoodherbs.com/Yarrow.html>
20. Moore, Michael. "Yarrow." *Medicinal Plants of the Pacific West.* Santa Fe, NM: Red Crane Books, 1993. Pages 272-275.
21. Herbs2000. "Yarrow Achillea millefolium." January 29, 2017. Web. <http://www.herbs2000.com/herbs/herbs_yarrow.htm>
22. Moore, Michael. "Yarrow." *Medicinal Plants of the Pacific West.* Santa Fe, NM: Red Crane Books, 1993. Pages 272-275.
23. Herbs2000. "Yarrow Achillea millefolium." January 29, 2017. Web. <http://www.herbs2000.com/herbs/herbs_yarrow.htm>
24. Whelan, Richard. "Yarrow." January 30, 2017. Web. <http://www.rjwhelan.co.nz/herbs%20A-Z/yarrow.html>
25. Gladstar, Rosemary. "Yarrow *Achillea millefolium* Compositae Parts Used: Leaves and Flowers." *Herbal Healing for Women: Simple Home Remedies for Women of All Ages.* New York, NY: Fireside, 1993. Pages 259-260.
26. Gladstar, Rosemary. "Yarrow *Achillea millefolium* Compositae Parts Used: Leaves and Flowers." *Herbal Healing for Women: Simple Home Remedies for Women of All Ages.* New York, NY: Fireside, 1993. Pages 259-260.
27. A Wandering Botanist: Tales of a lover of plants, history and travel, "Plant Story-- Yarrow, Achillea millefolium, an Ancient Healing Herb." <http://khkeeler.blogspot.com/2014/04/plant-story-yarrow-achillea-millefolium_6.html > Sunday, April 6, 2014   researched January 29, 2017
28. Gladstar, Rosemary. "Yarrow *Achillea millefolium* Compositae Parts Used: Leaves and Flowers." *Herbal Healing for Women: Simple Home Remedies for Women of All Ages.* New York, NY: Fireside, 1993. Pages 259-260.
29. Keeler, Kathleen. "Yarrow, Achillea millefolium, an Ancient Healing Herb." *A Wandering Botanist.* January 29, 2017. Web. <http://khkeeler.blogspot.com/2014/04/plant-story-yarrow-achillea-millefolium_6.html>
30. I Ching with Clarity. "I Ching Consultation: Yarrow or Coin? Some history." January 29, 2017. Web. <https://www.onlineclarity.co.uk/learn/ways-to-consult-the-i-ching/yarrow-or-coin>
31. Anthony, Carol, and Hanna Moog. "The Purpose of Consulting the I Ching Oracle." January 29, 2017. Web. <http://www.ichingoracle.com/our-blog/2017/2/22/article-4-the-purpose-of-consulting-the-i-ching-oracle-by-carol-and-hanna>

YELLOW DOCK

1. Return to Nature. "Harvesting Wild Docks." July 26, 2016. Web. <returntonature.us/stalking-the-curly-dock_rumex-crispus >
2. Thayer, Samuel. "Dock." *Nature's Garden: A Guide to Identifying, Harvesting, and Preparing Edible Wild Plants.* Birchwood, WI: Forager's Harvest Press, 2010. 226-237.
3. Global Healing Center. "What are the Benefits of Yellow Dock Root?" July 26, 2016. Web. <http://www.globalhealingcenter.com/natural-health/benefits-of-yellow-dock-root>
4. Global Healing Center. "What are the Benefits of Yellow Dock Root?" July 26, 2016. Web. <http://www.globalhealingcenter.com/natural-health/benefits-of-yellow-dock-root>
5. Global Healing Center. "What are the Benefits of Yellow Dock Root?" July 26, 2016. Web. <http://www.globalhealingcenter.com/natural-health/benefits-of-yellow-dock-root>
6. Global Healing Center. "What are the Benefits of Yellow Dock Root?" July 26, 2016. Web. <http://www.globalhealingcenter.com/natural-health/benefits-of-yellow-dock-root>
7. Skenderi, Gazmund. *Herbal Vade Mecum.* Rutherford, New Jersey: Herbacy Press, 2003.

8.   Return to Nature. "Harvesting Wild Docks." July 26, 2016. Web. <returntonature.us/stalking-the-curly-dock_rumex-crispus >
9.   Skenderi, Gazmund. *Herbal Vade Mecum.* Rutherford, New Jersey: Herbacy Press, 2003.
10.   Plants For A Future. "Rumex Crispus-L." July 26, 2016. Web. <pfaf.org/usure/plant.aspx? Latin name=RumexCrispus>
11.   Skenderi, Gazmund. *"Herbal Vade Mecum."* Rutherford, New Jersey: Herbacy Press, 2003.
12.   Plants for a Future. "Rumex Crispus-L." July 26, 2016. Web. <pfaf.org/usure/plant.aspx? Latin name=RumexCrispus>
13.   Return to Nature. "Harvesting Wild Docks." July 26, 2016. Web. <returntonature.us/stalking-the-curly-dock_rumex-crispus >
14.   Global Healing Center. "What are the Benefits of Yellow Dock Root?" July 26, 2016. Web. <http://www.globalhealingcenter.com/natural-health/benefits-of-yellow-dock-root>
15.   Plants For A Future. "Rumex Crispus-L." July 26, 2016. Web. <pfaf.org/usure/plant.aspx? Latin name=RumexCrispus>
16.   Return to Nature. "Harvesting Wild Docks." July 26, 2016. Web. <returntonature.us/stalking-the-curly-dock_rumex-crispus >
17.   Animal Man Survivor. "Wild Edible Plants: Curly Dock Leaves." July 26, 2016. Web. <youtube.com/watch?v-9nivATdDEVW>
18.   The Ohio State University. "Curly Dock." *Ohio Perennial and Biennial Weed Guide.* July 26, 2016. Web. <oardc.ohio-state.edu/weedguide/single_weed.phpid-39>
19.   The Ohio State University. "Curly Dock." *Ohio Perennial and Biennial Weed Guide.* July 26, 2016. Web. <oardc.ohio-state.edu/weedguide/single_weed.phpid-39>
20.   Plants For A Future. "Rumex Crispus-L." July 26, 2016. Web. <pfaf.org/usure/plant.aspx? Latin name=RumexCrispus>

OTHER SOURCES:
Middle Path Natural Health. "Yellow Dock: Rumex Crispus Health Uses." July 26, 2016. Web. <middlepath.com.au/plant/yellow-dock_rumex-crispus_potent-blood-tonic-purifier-tea-tincture.php>
Grieve, Mrs. M. "Docks." July 26, 2016. Web. <botanical.com/botanical/mgmh/d/docks-15.html>
Animal Man Survivor. "Wild Edible Plants: Curly Dock Leaves." July 26, 2016. Web. <youtube.com/watch?v-9nivATdDEVW>

YERBA BUENA

1.   "Can You Use Yerba Buena for Stomachaches?" December 28, 2015. Web. <livestrong.com/article/228187-the-yerba-buena-herb-for-stomachaches>
2.   "Can You Use Yerba Buena for Stomachaches?" December 28, 2015. Web. <livestrong.com/article/228187-the-yerba-buena-herb-for-stomachaches>
3.   "Can You Use Yerba Buena for Stomachaches?" December 28, 2015. Web. <livestrong.com/article/228187-the-yerba-buena-herb-for-stomachaches>
4.   Knoji. "Yerba Buena Herb: Medicinal Uses Aid Many Types of Pain Including Tooth Pain, Stomach Issues and Headaches." January 1, 2017. Web. <https://alternative-medicine.knoji.com/yerba-buena-herb-medicinal-uses-aid-many-types-of-pain-including-tooth-pain-stomach-issues-and-headaches>
5.   Moore, Michael. "Yerba Buena," *Medicinal Plants of the Pacific West,* Santa Fe, NM: Red Crane Books, 1993. Pages 278-280.
6.   Knoji. "Yerba Buena Herb: Medicinal Uses Aid Many Types of Pain Including Tooth Pain, Stomach Issues and Headaches." January 1, 2017. Web. <https://alternative-medicine.knoji.com/yerba-buena-herb-medicinal-uses-aid-many-types-of-pain-including-tooth-pain-stomach-issues-and-headaches>
7.   "Yerba Buena Micromeria chamissonis." December 28, 2015. Web. <naturalmedincalherbs.net/herbs/m/micromeria-chamissonis=yerba-buena.php>
8.   "Yerba Buena Micromeria chamissonis." December 28, 2015. Web. <naturalmedincalherbs.net/herbs/m/micromeria-chamissonis=yerba-buena.php>
9.   "The Good Herb Yerba Buena." <sparkletack.com/2007/12/01/the-good-herb-yerba-buena>
10.   "The good herb"yerba Buena." December 1, 2017 <sparkletack.com/2007/12/01/the-good-herb-yerba-buena>
11.   Knoji. "Yerba Buena Herb: Medicinal Uses Aid Many Types of Pain Including Tooth Pain, Stomach Issues and Headaches." January 1, 2017. Web. <https://alternative-medicine.knoji.com/yerba-buena-herb-medicinal-uses-aid-many-types-of-pain-including-tooth-pain-stomach-issues-and-headaches>
12.   Las Pilitas Nursery. "Satureja douglasii Yerba Buena." March 21, 2017. Web. <http://www.laspilitas.com/nature-of-california/plants/622--satureja-douglasii>
13.   United States Department of Agriculture, Natural Resources Conservation Service. *"Clinopodium douglasii* Yerba Buena." March 21, 2017. Web. <https://plants.usda.gov/core/profile?symbol=cldo2>

YERBA SANTA

1.   Skenderi, Gazmund. *Herbal Vade Mecum.* Rutherford, New Jersey: Herbacy Press, 2003.

.. Moore, Michael. "Yerba Santa." *Medicinal Plants of the Pacific West*. Santa Fe, NM: Red Crane Books, 1993. Pages 285-288.

. Moore, Michael. "Yerba Santa." *Medicinal Plants of the Pacific West*. Santa Fe, NM: Red Crane Books, 1993. Pages 285-288.

4. Skenderi, Gazmund. *Herbal Vade Mecum*. Rutherford, New Jersey: Herbacy Press, 2003.

5. Moore, Michael. "Yerba Santa." *Medicinal Plants of the Pacific West*. Santa Fe, NM: Red Crane Books, 1993. Pages 285-288.

5. Skenderi, Gazmund. *Herbal Vade Mecum*. Rutherford, New Jersey: Herbacy Press, 2003.

7. Skenderi, Gazmund. *Herbal Vade Mecum*. Rutherford, New Jersey: Herbacy Press, 2003.

8. Moore, Michael. "Yerba Santa." *Medicinal Plants of the Pacific West*. Santa Fe, NM: Red Crane Books, 1993. Pages 285-288.

9. Skenderi, Gazmund. *Herbal Vade Mecum*. Rutherford, New Jersey: Herbacy Press, 2003.

10. Moore, Michael. "Yerba Santa." *Medicinal Plants of the Pacific West*. Santa Fe, NM: Red Crane Books, 1993. Pages 285-288.

11. Indian Mirror. "Yerba Santa." December 20, 2016. Web. <http://www.indianmirror.com/ayurveda/yerba-santa.html>

12. Indian Mirror. "Yerba Santa." December 20, 2016. Web. <http://www.indianmirror.com/ayurveda/yerba-santa.html>

13. Indian Mirror. "Yerba Santa." December 20, 2016. Web. <http://www.indianmirror.com/ayurveda/yerba-santa.html>

14. Indian Mirror. "Yerba Santa." December 20, 2016. Web. <http://www.indianmirror.com/ayurveda/yerba-santa.html>

RECIPES

BASIC INTERNAL RECIPES

1. "Herbal Infusions and Decoctions – Preparing Medicinal Teas." *Chestnut School of Herbal Medicine*, April 15, 2017. Web. <chestnutherbs.com/herbal-infusions-and-decoctions-preparing-medicinal-teas>

2. Gladstar, Rosemary. *Herbal Healing for Women: Simple Home Remedies for Women of All Ages*. New York, NY: Fireside, 1993. Print.

3. Gladstar, Rosemary. *Herbal Healing for Women: Simple Home Remedies for Women of All Ages*. New York, NY: Fireside, 1993. Print.

4. "Herbal Infusions and Decoctions – Preparing Medicinal Teas." *Chestnut School of Herbal Medicine*, April 15, 2017. Web. <chestnutherbs.com/herbal-infusions-and-decoctions-preparing-medicinal-teas>

5. Gladstar, Rosemary. *Herbal Healing for Women: Simple Home Remedies for Women of All Ages*. New York, NY: Fireside, 1993. Print.

6. "Herbal Infusions and Decoctions – Preparing Medicinal Teas." *Chestnut School of Herbal Medicine*, April 15, 2017. Web. <chestnutherbs.com/herbal-infusions-and-decoctions-preparing-medicinal-teas>

7. Gladstar, Rosemary. *Herbal Healing for Women: Simple Home Remedies for Women of All Ages*. New York, NY: Fireside, 1993. Print.

8. Gladstar, Rosemary. *Herbal Healing for Women: Simple Home Remedies for Women of All Ages*. New York, NY: Fireside, 1993. Print.

9. "Herbal Infusions and Decoctions – Preparing Medicinal Teas." *Chestnut School of Herbal Medicine*, April 15, 2017. Web. <chestnutherbs.com/herbal-infusions-and-decoctions-preparing-medicinal-teas>

10. Gladstar, Rosemary. *Herbal Healing for Women: Simple Home Remedies for Women of All Ages*. New York, NY: Fireside, 1993. Print.

11. Gladstar, Rosemary. *Herbal Healing for Women: Simple Home Remedies for Women of All Ages*. New York, NY: Fireside, 1993. Print.

12. Gladstar, Rosemary. *Herbal Healing for Women: Simple Home Remedies for Women of All Ages*. New York, NY: Fireside, 1993. Print.

13. "How To Make Herbal Syrups." *Mountain rose herbs.com*, April 15, 2016. <https://blog.mountainroseherbs.com/homemade-herbal-syrups>

14. "How To Make Herbal Syrups." *Mountain rose herbs.com*, April 15, 2016. <https://blog.mountainroseherbs.com/homemade-herbal-syrups>

SPECIFIC INTERNAL RECIPES

1. Blue Elderberry Syrup: "Intermediate Herbal Course." *Herbal Academy of New England*, May 27, 2017. Web. <members.herbalacademyofne.com/course/intermediate-herbal-course>

2. Harvesting and Preparing Giant Kelp: Drum, Ryan. "Sea Vegetables for Food and Medicine." *Island herbs*, May 28, 2017. Web. <ryandrum.com/seaxpan1.html>

BASIC EXTERNAL RECIPES

1. Gladstar, Rosemary. *Herbal Healing for Women: Simple Home Remedies for Women of All Ages*. New York, NY: Fireside, 1993. Print.

2. Moore, Michael. *Medicinal Plants of the Pacific West*. Santa Fe, NM: Red Crane Books, 1993. Print.

3.   "Intermediate Herbal Course." *Herbal Academy of New England,* May 27, 2017. Web.
      <members.herbalacademyofne.com/course/intermediate-herbal-course>
4.   "Poultice vs compress." *Mockingbird Meadows Farm.* April 3, 2017. Web.
      <mockingbirdmeadows.com/2012/10/15/poultice-vs-compress>
5.   "Poultice vs. Compress vs. Fomentation… What's the difference?" *Basic Home Medicine,* April 3, 2017.
      Web. <basichomemedicine.wordpress.com/2013/07/15/poultice-vs-compress-vs-fomentation-whats-
      the-difference>
6.   "Poultice vs compress." *Mockingbird Meadows Farm.* April 3, 2017. Web.
      <mockingbirdmeadows.com/2012/10/15/poultice-vs-compress>
7.   "Poultice vs compress." *Mockingbird Meadows Farm.* April 3, 2017. Web.
      <mockingbirdmeadows.com/2012/10/15/poultice-vs-compress>
8.   "Poultice vs. Compress vs. Fomentation… What's the difference?" *Basic Home Medicine,* April 3, 2017.
      Web. <basichomemedicine.wordpress.com/2013/07/15/poultice-vs-compress-vs-fomentation-whats-
      the-difference>
9.   "Natural Healing: Herbal Bath Delights." *Mother Earth Living: Natural Home, Healthy Life,* April 5, 2017.
      Web.< motherearthliving.com/Health-and-Wellness/natural-healing-herbal-bath-
      delights?pageid=2#PageContent2>
10.   "Natural Healing: Herbal Bath Delights." *Mother Earth Living: Natural Home, Healthy Life,* April 5, 2017.
      Web.< motherearthliving.com/Health-and-Wellness/natural-healing-herbal-bath-
      delights?pageid=2#PageContent2>
11.   "Natural Healing: Herbal Bath Delights." *Mother Earth Living: Natural Home, Healthy Life,* April 5, 2017.
      Web.< motherearthliving.com/Health-and-Wellness/natural-healing-herbal-bath-
      delights?pageid=2#PageContent2>
12.   Robertsdottir, Anna R. *Icelandic Herbs and Their Medicinal Uses,* April 4, 2017. Berkeley, CA: North
      Atlantic Books, 2013. Google books.
      <https://books.google.com/books?id=cx3XCwAAQBAJ&pg=PA10&lpg=PA10&dq=medicinalherb
      +gargles&source=bl&ots=bt8gtojGEZ&sig=dtMTsMscQbRELKdOL5rbO85DLos&hl=en&sa=X&
      ved=0ahUKEwjMzPzXqozTAhWnj1QKHcpMCF0Q6AEIJDAB#v=onepage&q=medicinal%20herb
      %20gargles&f=false>

SPECIFIC EXTERNAL RECIPES

1.   Himalayan Blackberry Astringent: Falconi, Dina. *Earthly Bodies & Heavenly Hair.* Woodstock, NY:
      Ceres Press, 1998. Print.

ABOUT THE AUTHOR AND ILLUSTRATOR

Levi Glatt is a Cabrillo College student and homeschooler who enjoys wildcrafting and exploring the breathtaking natural landscapes of Santa Cruz, California. After months of dedicated study, Levi received an Intermediate Herbal Certificate from the International School of Herbal Arts and Sciences.

From a young age, Levi has expressed a deep passion for plants. As a toddler, he began learning how to recognize edible plants, teaching relatives how to identify his favorites, Pineapple Weed and Sour Grass.

Levi's artwork has been published in *Highlights*, a magazine with over two million readers, as well as the *Santa Cruz Sentinel*. He has received numerous awards for his art and photography at the Santa Cruz County Fair, including Best of Section.

Levi is appreciative of the opportunity and resources to learn about medicinal plants to a greater extent. He is thankful for the research that often dates back thousands of years, and is grateful for the beautiful environment where we can discover them growing all around us.

Made in the USA
San Bernardino, CA
27 September 2018